Bearing Witness to the Witness

Bearing Witness to the Witness examines different modes of traumatic testimony and the ways in which these modes can enrich or undermine the ability of the subject to bear witness. Years of listening to both direct and indirect testimonies on trauma has led Dana Amir to identify four modes of witnessing trauma: the "metaphoric mode", the "metonymic mode", the "excessive mode" and the "*Muselmann* mode".

To follow these four modes of interaction with the traumatic memory, the various chapters of the book present a close reading of three genres of traumatic witnessing: literary accounts by Holocaust survivors, memoirs (located between autobiographic recollection and fiction) and "raw" testimonies taken from Holocaust survivors. Since every traumatic testimonial narrative contains a combination of all four modes with various shifts between them, it is of crucial importance to identify the singular combination of modes that characterizes each traumatic narrative, focusing on the specific areas within which a shift occurs from one mode to another. Such a focus is extremely important, as illustrated and analyzed throughout this book, to the rehabilitation of the psychic metabolic system which conditions the digestion of traumatic materials, allowing a metaphoric working through of traumatic zones that were so far only accessible to repetition and evacuation.

Bearing Witness to the Witness will appeal to trauma researchers of all research areas, including psychologists, psychoanalysts, literary scholars, as well as philosophers of language and philosophers of the mind. The book will also be of interest and relevance to clinical psychologists, psychoanalytic candidates and graduate students in literary theory and criticism.

Dana Amir is Faculty member at Haifa University, a clinical psychologist, training and supervising psychoanalyst at the Israel Psychoanalytic Society, poetess and literature researcher. She is the author of six poetry books and two psychoanalytic books, and the winner of many national as well as four distinguished international prizes. Her papers have been published in many journals and presented in professional conferences all over the world.

'Taking Dana Amir's approach as a model, a new line of inquiry, that of reconstructing the mental processes that led to the phenomena observed in the testimonies, will become evident, leading to a much deeper understanding of the experience of survival and of its aftermath. Her book is written in a prose that is almost poetry and in a language that is both strong as well as daring and imaginative.'

Professor Dori Laub, Clinical Professor of Psychiatry,
Yale University School of Medicine, USA

When music is played in a new key, the melody does not change, but the notes that make up the composition do: change in the context of continuity, a continuity that perseveres through change. Psychoanalysis in a New Key publishes books that share the aims psychoanalysts have always had, but that approach them differently. The books in the series are not expected to advance any particular theoretical agenda, although to this date most have been written by analysts from the Interpersonal and Relational orientations.

The most important contribution of a psychoanalytic book is the communication of something that nudges the reader's grasp of clinical theory and practice in an unexpected direction. Psychoanalysis in a New Key creates a deliberate focus on innovative and unsettling clinical thinking. Because that kind of thinking is encouraged by exploration of the sometimes surprising contributions to psychoanalysis of ideas and findings from other fields, Psychoanalysis in a New Key particularly encourages interdisciplinary studies. Books in the series have married psychoanalysis with dissociation, trauma theory, sociology and criminology. The series is open to the consideration of studies examining the relationship between psychoanalysis and any other field – for instance, biology, literary and art criticism, philosophy, systems theory, anthropology and political theory.

But innovation also takes place within the boundaries of psychoanalysis, and Psychoanalysis in a New Key therefore also presents work that reformulates thought and practice without leaving the precincts of the field. Books in the series focus, for example, on the significance of personal values in psychoanalytic practice, on the complex interrelationship between the analyst's clinical work and personal life, on the consequences for the clinical situation when patient and analyst are from different cultures, and on the need for psychoanalysts to accept the degree to which they knowingly satisfy their own wishes during treatment hours, often to the patient's detriment. A full list of all titles in this series is available at: https://www.routledge.com/series/LEAPNKBS

TITLES IN THIS SERIES INCLUDE:

Vol. 47 Bearing Witness to the Witness
A Psychoanalytic Perspective on Four Modes of Traumatic Testimony
Dana Amir

Vol. 46 Travels with the Self
Interpreting Psychology as Cultural History
Philip Cushman

Bearing Witness to the Witness

A Psychoanalytic Perspective on Four Modes of Traumatic Testimony

Dana Amir

Routledge
Taylor & Francis Group
LONDON AND NEW YORK

First published 2019
by Routledge
2 Park Square, Milton Park, Abingdon, Oxon OX14 4RN

and by Routledge
711 Third Avenue, New York, NY 10017

Routledge is an imprint of the Taylor & Francis Group, an informa business

British Library Cataloguing-in-Publication Data
A catalogue record for this book is available from the British Library

Library of Congress Cataloging-in-Publication Data
Names: Amir, Dana, author.
Title: Bearing witness to the witness: a psychoanalytic perspective on four modes of traumatic testimony/Dana Amir.
Description: Abingdon, Oxon; New York, NY: Routledge, 2019. | Series: Psychoanalysis in a new key book series; 47 | Includes bibliographical references and index.
Identifiers: LCCN 2018025202 (print) | LCCN 2018037264 (ebook) | ISBN 9781315146508 (Master) | ISBN 9781351379489 (Web PDF) | ISBN 9781351379472 (ePub) | ISBN 9781351379465 (Mobipocket/Kindle) | ISBN 9781138505292 (hardback: alk. paper) | ISBN 9781138505308 (pbk.: alk. paper) | ISBN 9781315146508 (ebk.)
Subjects: LCSH: Psychic trauma–Treatment. | Holocaust survivors–Psychology.
Classification: LCC RC552.T7 (ebook) | LCC RC552.T7 A46 2019 (print) | DDC 616.85/210651–dc23
LC record available at https://lccn.loc.gov/2018025202

ISBN: 978-1-138-50529-2 (hbk)
ISBN: 978-1-138-50530-8 (pbk)
ISBN: 978-1-315-14650-8 (ebk)

Typeset in Times New Roman
by by Deanta Global Publishing Services, Chennai, India

To my family, lost and found

Contents

Acknowledgments

I would like to express my deepest gratitude to the editor of this series, Donnell Stern, for enabling such a space for psychoanalytic thinking outside the scale; to Professor Dori Laub, who was for me and for many others a source of unique inspiration, and to Mirjam Hadar for her excellent linguistic editing.

This book is based on a research supported by The Israel Science Foundation (grant No. 679/13).

Every effort has been made to contact the copyright holders for their permission to reprint selections of this book. The publishers would be grateful to hear from any copyright holder who is not here acknowledged and will undertake to rectify any errors or omissions in future editions of this book.

Selected parts from Chapter 1 and Chapter 8 were first published in the following paper and reprinted by permission of Taylor & Francis, LLC:

Amir, D. (2016). When language meets the traumatic lacuna: The metaphoric, the metonymic and the psychotic modes of testimony. *Psychoanalytic Inquiry*, 36(8), 620–632, DOI: 10.1080/07351690.2016.1226045. This paper was also selected as the winner of the IPA (International Psychoanalytic Association) Hayman prize (2017).

Selected parts from Chapter 2 were first published in the following paper and reprinted by permission of *fort da*:

Amir, D. (2017). Traumatic miss and the work of mourning. *fort da*, 23(2), 7–16.

Selected parts from Chapter 2 were first also published in the following chapter and reprinted by permission of Cambridge Scholars Publishing House:

Amir, D. (2018). Autobiographical fiction or fictive autobiography? Georges Perec's unique mode of traumatic testimony. In: *Trauma and literature*. UK: Cambridge Scholars Publishing House.

Selected parts from Chapter 7 were first published in the following paper and reprinted by permission of *American Imago*:

Amir, D. (2018). From the collapse of signifiers to the reconstruction of language: Robert Antelme's *The human race*. *American Imago*.

Selected parts from Chapter 8 were first published in the following paper and reprinted by permission of *Psychoanalytic Quarterly*:

Amir, D. (2018). Awakening to and from the traumatic lacuna. *The Psychoanalytic Quarterly*, 87(2), 303–321.

Selected parts from Chapter 10 were first published in the following paper and reprinted with permission of Guilford Press:

Amir, D. (2016). Hermetic narratives and false analysis: A unique variant of the mechanism of identification with the aggressor. *The Psychoanalytic Review*, 103(4), 539–549.

Literary quotations from *The Human Race* by Robert Antelme were reprinted with the permission of Editions Gallimard, Paris and the Marlboro press, Marlboro Vermont. Originally published in French in 1957 under the title *L'espèce humaine*. Copyright © 1957 by Éditions Gallimard, Paris. First published in English in 1992 by The Marlboro Press, Marlboro, Vermont. Translation copyright © 1992 by Jeffrey Haight and Annie Mahler. The Marlboro Press/Northwestern Edition published 1998 by arrangement with Editions Gallimard. All rights reserved.

Literary quotations from "Bertha" by Aharon Appelfeld were reprinted with the permission of The Wylie Agency (UK) Limited. English translation Copyright © Institute for the Translation of Hebrew Literature. First published in Israel 1965. Published by arrangement with The Institute for the Translation of Hebrew Literature

Literary quotations from Georges Perec's *W, or the Memory of Childhood* trans. David Bellos are reprinted by permission of David R. Godine, Publisher, Inc. Copyright © Georges Perec, 1987.

Literary quotations from Ida Fink's short stories were reprinted with the permission of Peter Owen Publishers, UK.

Excerpt from *The Notebook* copyright © 1988 by Alan Sheridan. Used by permission of Grove/Atlantic, Inc. Any third party use of this material, outside of this publication, is prohibited.

Foreword

Dori Laub

The number of testimonies obtained and recorded from Holocaust survivors by now probably exceeds 100,000 and they are preserved in archives and libraries in many countries of the world. There is a very large discrepancy however between the extraordinary depth and richness we attribute to the material contained in the testimonies and the amount of attention and study it has given rise to. Only a fraction of the testimonies have been watched and even fewer have been studied. Family members, including second and third generations, are reluctant to view them and researchers find it difficult to work with them. They do not know what the relevant questions are to properly address the testimonial material or what methodologies to use to probe its depth while evaluating it. In other words, we lack the tools with which we could carry out meaningful work with this very rich and extraordinarily valuable database.

To this end, Dana Amir's present book constitutes a major contribution. Proceeding from a theory of testimony – "that testimony is always the attempt to bear witness to something that failed to be registered as it happened, and its modalities represent various types of awakenings to this failure", she continues to elaborate that often an all-engulfing traumatic lacunae comes to replace such failed registrations and consequently absent memories. She draws from Georgio Agamben's observation that there are two Latin words for the English word "witness". The first is "testis" – the mediator, the third party in the conflict between two sides. The other word is "supertestis" – the one having experienced something to its ultimate end, can testify to it. The Holocaust survivor's inner witness shifts between these two meanings: having undergone the full experience, he also functions as the "testis", the mediator between the ultimate experience and language. The above-mentioned modalities of testimony that she formulates, are four: the metaphorical mode, in which self-reflection and the creation of new meaning, movement and memory exist, on the one hand; and the metonymic, the excessive and the Muselmann modes, which are essentially non-mentalized reenactments of the experience, on the other.

Dana Amir elaborates on and fleshes out the different new concepts she introduces in great detail and in depth, both in her testimonial and in her literary examples. She treats both texts – the testimonial and the literary as if they where clinical material and applies clinical concepts such as defense, dissociation, identity, self, the reflective I, etc., in her analysis of both of them. She freely and creatively uses her own imagination, that is her countertransference responses, in deepening that analysis and bringing it to closure. Reading the book, future researchers will become thoroughly familiar with the new concepts and will make use of them in working with testimonies. They will know how to view testimonies, what to look for and what questions to ask of themselves. They will become cognizant of the criteria that apply in studying and categorizing the testimonies. Taking Dana Amir's approach as a model, a new line of inquiry, that of reconstructing the mental processes that led to the phenomena observed in the testimonies, will become evident, leading to a much deeper understanding of the experience of survival and of its aftermath.

The book is written in a prose that is almost poetry and in a language that is both strong as well as daring and imaginative.

Introduction

My grandmother was the youngest of three children in a family from Lvov, Poland, which, except her, was killed in its entirety during the Holocaust. The younger of her two older brothers was called Shammai. Shemeck. For many of the years of long life after the Holocaust she would have the same dream about him: together they board the train headed most likely for Auschwitz. The train suddenly stops, and she jumps off, thinking he is behind her, only to realize a moment later that he has remained on board. Then she wakes up.

In actuality, she came to Palestine shortly before the Second World War and the scene in the dream never occurred. A German soldier shot dead her brother one evening in the street near his house, a few weeks before the entire family was sent to the concentration camps. Yet the dream repeated itself over and over again throughout the years. A few months before her death she told me she had had the same dream again, but this time it was slightly different: She boards the train with Shemeck, the train arrives at the place where in her usual dream she jumps off, but this time she stays on board with him.

When she told me this dream I thought it portended her approaching death, and therefore understood the change in the dream plot as a replacement of the wish to unite her life with his life – with the wish that her death would be united with his death. During the writing of this book, however, something else occurred to me: staying on the train represented not only the wish to reunite with him. It was, in Cathy Caruth's (1996) terminology, an attempt to undo the awakening from the dream, which is in effect waking up to the missing of the traumatic event of separation. It was not the wish to take him off the train along with her that motivated the recurrent dream, but rather the wish to get back on the train to catch up with the moment when she failed to notice that he had remained on board.

In this sense, the dream was an act of bearing witness: bearing witness to a moment of inattention; bearing witness to the blind spot which held the great loss that went on haunting her throughout her life and to which she awakened only a moment too late. The recurrence of the dream was related not only to her guilt at not having saved him or at not having died together with him, but also, to the randomness of her own survival. It referred to the arbitrary, absent-minded moment that separated her leap off the train from his staying on it, or maybe to the arbitrary moment that was the actual referent of this dream – the moment that made all the difference between her almost random decision to leave Poland and his decision to stay behind. The recurrence of the dream was related therefore not only to her survivor's guilt, but also, to her attempt to claim her survival – which she experienced as accidental and arbitrary: to claim it as an event that belonged to her and with which she could identify (Amir, 2017).

In the introduction to *Remnants of Auschwitz* (2002) Agamben writes:

> At a certain point, it became clear that testimony contained at its core an essential lacuna; in other words, the survivors bore witness to something that it is impossible to bear witness to. As a consequence, commenting on survivors' testimony necessarily meant interrogating this lacuna, or more precisely, attempting to listen to it.
>
> (ibid., p. 13)

This book directs attention to the lacuna that constitutes the capacity to bear witness and at the same time undermines it. Years of listening to both direct and indirect testimonies on trauma have led me to identify four modes of witnessing, reflecting four modes in which language collapses into the traumatic lacuna: the "metaphoric mode", the "metonymic mode", the "excessive mode" and the "*Muselmann* mode". These four modes of witnessing are distinguished by the degree of psychic motility they succeed to form in relation to traumatic memories. The most developed mode, which I call the metaphoric mode of witnessing, imitates the analogous movement that metaphor creates in language, simultaneously holding two frames of reference: that of the victim (the experiencing I) and that of the witness (the narrating I). The other three modes (the metonymic, the excessive and the *Muselmann* modes) gradually decline in terms of their capacity to hold the traumatic memories in mind in a way that allows for transformation.

To follow these four modes of interaction with the traumatic object, the next chapters will present a close-reading of three genres of traumatic witnessing: the first of these are literary accounts written mostly by Holocaust survivors. The works discussed under this category are *W, or the Memory of Childhood* by George Perec, *The Notebook* by Agota Kristóf, *House of Dolls* by Ka-Tzetnik, six short stories by Ida Fink and the short story "Bertha" by Aharon Appelfeld. The second genre, located between autobiographic recollection and fiction, is memoir. The work at the center of my discussion of this category is Robert Antelme's *The Human Race*. The third genre are "raw" testimonies taken from Holocaust survivors, which were sampled from two archives: an archive of children-survivors' testimonies which were documented right after the war, and an archive of testimonies of survivors who were children during the war but were interviewed in depth only many years later. Behind this choice was the assumption that the comparison between the three genres is in fact a comparison between three degrees of distancing; while the oral testimonies could be thought of as having undergone the least degree of working through, reflecting thereby only minor (if any) distancing from the "gross traumatic experience", I considered the memoir to represent at least a certain degree of distancing from the traumatic experience. Along similar lines, I assumed that since the literary testimonies underwent the highest degree of aesthetic, intellectual and emotional elaboration, they would constitute the most distanced accounts. Assuming these three levels of distancing, I assumed that the most metaphoric mode would then be manifest in the literary testimonies, while the most psychotic manifestations were likely to occur in the raw testimonies. This, however, was rarely the case. Each individual representative of a genre revealed a rich and complex fabric consisting of all four modes in varying degrees of dominance. These singular weavings of the modes into one another within every genre, and again within every single narrative, portraying diverse and wondrous mindsets and manifesting unique relations between traumatic lacunae and modes of transcendence – illustrate, I believe, not only various ways of coping with trauma, but also the unique modes by which the human psyche claims possession, and re-constitutes itself by means of this claiming.

Consideration of the expressly literary works introduced me to an additional, critical layer of analysis. Of the three genres discussed in this book, this is the only one in which there is a built-in gap between two aspects of bearing witness: the standpoint of the literary protagonist and that of the author who is not identical to this protagonist even when his or her writing is declaredly autobiographical. This structural distance between protagonist and author creates, in effect, a metaphoric gap. This gap is neither always present in the text itself – which at times, as I will demonstrate, may be written in an excessive or a metonymic mode – nor is it always located in the reader's countertransference to the text. The gap results, rather, from the simple non-identity between the writer and his or her protagonist. One can say, then, that the genre of literary testimony – even when that testimony is psychotic in its mode or creates a metonymic reenactment in the reader response – enables metaphoric distancing.

"'Ego' is he who says 'ego'", argued the linguist Emile Benveniste (1971, p. 24): the narrator constitutes himself through the narrative. The space between "ego" ("the subject of utterance") and narrator ("the subject of enunciation") is precisely the space that enables the shift necessary for bearing witness, and not only in the literary act. For in order to become a witness it is necessary at times to leave the subject of utterance on one side of language as the subject of enunciation crosses to the other side. In the testimonial text, the subject of utterance does not necessarily coincide with the subject of enunciation. They may remain on either side of the traumatic event, sometimes tied to one another in the most tenuous of ways. In the non-literary testimonies as in the literary works, one may identify moments in which the subject of utterance and the subject of enunciation engage in lively dialogue, as well as moments when the gap between them cannot be bridged, and those in which they both collapse, each into the abyss of the other side. But due to the space it assumes between protagonist and narrator, the very act of bearing witness offers a chance to create some movement in relation to a hitherto frozen, circular traumatic present.

I would like to return now to my grandmother's recurrent dream. The moment in which she loses her brother in that dream is not only marked by her turning away but also by a freezing in time. The train stops. This stop enables her to jump off, but also to turn her back on his loss. The dream in which she stays on the train erases this freezing in time and reconstitutes continuity and movement, even if it is a movement towards death. In this sense, it could also be understood as her last attempt to constitute her own life as a continuum, devoid of fragmentation, devoid of cessation. For on the train in that last dream the movement of life, however paradoxically, can no longer be halted.

References

Agamben, G. (2002). *Remnants of Auschwitz: The witness and the archive*. (trans: D. Heller-Roazen). New York: Zone Books.

Amir, D. (2017). Traumatic miss and the work of mourning. *fort da*, 23(2), 7–16.

Benveniste, E. ([1966] 1971). *Problems in general linguistics*. (trans: M.E. Meek). Coral Gables, FL: University of Miami Press.

Caruth, C. (1996). *Unclaimed experience: Trauma narrative and history*. Baltimore, MD: Johns Hopkins University Press.

Chapter 1

When language meets the traumatic lacuna

Four modes of traumatic testimony

Traumatic experiences often activate a psychic process of self-annihilation. Their acidity creates types of psychic holes that absorb the unbearable traumatic substances along with the subject who contains them, to the point of a total collapse of inner barriers. Paradoxically, this collapse of barriers leaves the subject imprisoned in a territory of *negative possession* (Amir, 2012, 2014), where the traumatic contents are neither digested nor worked through. The only chance of recovery from this condition lies in the possibility to deposit the traumatic substances in another subject who cannot be annihilated by them. This is the core of bearing witness.

The psychoanalytic literature on trauma refers extensively to the major role of the other in bearing witness to a trauma the victim often has not, and could not have, witnessed him or herself. Authors from various theoretical fields (Laub and Auerhahn, 1993; Oliner, 1996) describe trauma as something that has taken place "over there, far away", an event that does not belong to the experiencing "I". Trauma is often conceptualized as an external event, detached from the narrator who experienced it. Survivors of trauma claim that they live in two worlds: the world of their traumatic memories (a kind of everlasting present) and the real world (the concrete present). Usually they neither wish nor are able to integrate these two worlds. As a result, the traumatic memory is preserved frozen and timeless, and psychic movement becomes automatic, aimless and senseless (Laub, 2005).

At the heart of the traumatic experience there is an experience of excess that escapes representation and leaves a lacuna within consciousness (LaCapra, 2001). Caruth (1996, pp. 91–92) writes about the traumatic paradox in which the most direct contact with the violent event may occur only through the very inability to know it. Trauma is not only an experience, but also the failure to experience that experience; not merely the threat itself, but the fact that the threat was recognized as such only a moment too late. As it was not experienced in time, the event is condemned not to be fully known (Caruth, 1996, p. 62). As such, it returns to claim its presence, trying to cover an experiential void through compulsive repetition. Van der Kolk et al. (1996) argues that while terrifying events may be remembered extremely vividly, they may equally resist any kind of integration. These memories remain powerful but frozen, un-transformable by either circumstantial processes or the passing of time. They are subject to neither assimilation nor developmental change since they are not integrated into the associative network. As a result, they remain concealed, retaining their magnetic force in their detailed and contradictory clarity, in the condensed vagueness that envelopes them. Rather than undergoing the transformation that leads to a personal narrative, traumatic experiences are imprinted as primary impressions that do not receive verbal representation (ibid., pp. 282, 296). As Modell (2006) suggests, trauma tends to freeze the past and therefore "deprives it of the plasticity it needs if it is to connect to the present" (Stern, 2012, p. 56). Memories of trauma are not only rigid and concrete – but unmentalized. As such, they remain "things-in-themselves", neither adaptable nor generative (ibid.).

In her book *The Parents Who Live Through Me* (2010)[1] Yolanda Gampel describes the permanent co-existence, typical of Holocaust survivors and other victims of collective violence, of two "background images": one is a "background of security" and the other is a "background of the uncanny". According to Gampel, children whose parents died in the Holocaust witnessed the sudden erasure – physical as well as emotional – of their parents and were often left with alienated parental figures, frozen and lifeless. As a result, "a background of the uncanny" emerged (Gampel, 1999). From that point on, this background is the receptacle of all loss and functions, simultaneously, as its means of denial, likely to express itself in the form of "psychic holes". In a paper discussing the multi-faceted mutations of these traumatic encapsulations, Gampel and Mazor (2004) write:

> It is the real, das Ding, and the chaos. It breaks the narrative of life. It creates a semantic hole that doesn't fit in with the rest. It does not enter the continuum of biographical narrative, because new experiences stumble across a hole, a gap, a limit, and thus it cannot become a

> part of the continuum and cannot turn dialectic within the personality. A new uncanny background has been created, one that does not allow the experiences to enter the former background.
>
> (p. 555)

In a very similar context, Vivian Liska (2009) writes:

> For decades, literary approximations of silence determined the poetics of Holocaust remembrance. This poetics assumed that only silence can truly render what occurred and convey the horrors of this past in a language uncontaminated by inadequate discourse. Since the ultimate witness, the dead, are silent and speak only through the living, it is silence itself that is summoned. Only silence itself, the interruption of communicative speech, the empty space between words, the self-erasing trace of the non-representable, the open wound of the abyss, the caesura, the rupture, the stuttered, stammered word approaching silence, is true.
>
> (p. 151)

Dori Laub (2005), in a paper entitled "Traumatic Shutdown of Narrative and Symbolization", quotes Moore (1999) who argued that the traumatized subject cannot know that the traumatic event has taken place until another supplies it with a narrative. A person can know his or her story only when he or she tells it to what Laub calls "the inner thou" (internal other). But since trauma critically injures both the internal and external other – namely the addressee of any dialogical relationship – it ruins the possibility of an empathic dyad in the inner representation of the world, leaving the subject with nobody to address, either inside or outside him or herself.[2] This catastrophic loss of the good object compels the victim to internalize the only available object, the aggressor himself, as a malignant self-object (Kohut, 1971) with whom he or she identifies. Laub further argues that the fragmenting effects of the traumatic experience can be better understood if we postulate the presence of unbound, un-neutralized death instinct derivatives.[3] Conscious memory is the first casualty of these unbound death instinct derivatives. Furthermore, erasure of traumatically lost objects and of the traumatic experience itself may lead the survivor to complete oblivion, or to doubt the veracity and authenticity of his or her own experiences, compromising his or her entire sense of identity and continuity. Laub contends that it is the traumatic loss of the (internal) good object and the libidinal ties to it that releases the hitherto neutralized forces of the death instinct and intensifies the clinical manifestations of its derivatives. "In the absence of an internal responsive 'thou', there is no attachment to nor cathexis of the object" (Laub, 2005, pp. 316–317).

Shoshana Felman (1992) similarly reflects on Albert Camus's *The Plague* (2004):

> [The protagonist] has to learn on his body what a holocaust – a situation of "total condemnation" – is: [...] an experience that requires one to live through one's own death, and paradoxically, bear witness to that living through one's dying; a death experience which can be truly comprehended, witnessed only from inside (from inside the witness's own annihilation); a radical experience to which no outsider can be witness, but to which no witness can be, or remain, outsider.
>
> (p. 109)

Metaphoric, metonymic and psychotic modes of witnessing

Metaphor and metonymy are two forms of semantic shift, that is, two modes of transition from one semantic field to another. Metaphor is the use of a word or an expression in a borrowed, rather than in its simple original sense, or the use of the characteristics of one concept in order to illuminate another. Metaphor is based on analogy, on a relationship of similarity between two semantic fields. The sentence "my love is a rose" does not imply that the rose itself is the beloved one but that something in the beloved's features resembles those of a rose. Metonymy, by contrast, is a figurative tool that illustrates something by replacing it with something else that is situated close to it in time or space, or that belongs in the same context. The result is not logical in the simple sense and can only be understood through the proximity between the two elements. This is how the expression "the White House" comes to stand for the notion of "the President's spokesperson". As opposed to metaphor, in metonymy there is no transfer of characteristics between the two elements (the President's spokesperson does not share features with the White House). The connection between them is associative only in a way that allows us to perceive the one as representative of the other.

In his article "Two Aspects of Language and Two Types of Aphasic Disturbances" (1956), Roman Jakobson presents metaphor and metonymy as polar opposites rather than parts of the hierarchical order in which they are more commonly seen. He stresses the *similarity* metaphor installs between its signifiers versus the *contiguity* typical of metonymy. Each of these modes of transposition, he argues, relies on different cognitive skills. While metaphor is based on the cognitive ability to convert, metonymy implies the ability to connect and contextualize, that is, the ability to create continuity and to identify something as part of – and following from – a context. Jakobson divides the aphasic patients with whom his article is concerned into patients who suffer from impaired identification of similarities as opposed to those whose ability to combine and contextualize is affected.

Lacan's (1958, 1977) distinction between metaphor and metonymy diverges from Jakobson's. Though, following the latter, he associates metaphor with the axis of linguistic selection and metonymy with that of combination, metaphor for him acts to constitute meaning while metonymy resists meaning: the metonymic drive is related to the desire to recover the lost "Real". Metaphor, by contrast, is associated with "the symptom", whose creation is a constructive process in which new meaning emerges. Metaphor therefore maintains analogous relations between its subjects, while in metonymy subjects entertain relations of contiguous association. Metaphor is related to the ability to take a distance, thereby enabling the discussion of something that belongs to one conceptual field in terms that belong to another. Metonymy, by contrast, constitutes relations of continuity, that is relations that maintain no distance.

Following both Jakobson's and Lacan's ideas, I would like to suggest a distinction between a metaphoric and a metonymic mode of witnessing, further adding a psychotic mode (divided into two sub-modes) which is completely outside the range stretching between the former two.

The term "metaphoric mode of witnessing" refers to those parts of the testimonial narrative where there is a shift from the "first person" to the "third person" of experience, or from the *experiencing I* to the *reflective I*,[4] further enabling the shift from the "position of the victim" to the "position of the witness" (Amir, 2012, 2014, 2015, 2016). The metaphoric mode, by its very nature, creates movement and is based on movement. Unlike the other three modes which will be described later – the metaphoric mode struggles against traumatic stagnation through creating a three-dimensional space based on the shift from the first person to the third person and back. Its metaphoric quality lies therefore in the fact that it involves an act of representation and the creation of new meaning, producing an integrated narrative within which the traumatic events are not merely repeated but also undergo transformation.

As against the metaphoric mode, the metonymic mode of witnessing remains a "first person" mode of report. It produces a text that preserves and enacts the traumatic memories and the traumatic features and is thus characterized by the same sense of isolation, fragmentation, disorientation and lack of coherence that are typical of the traumatic experience itself. In that sense, the metonymic mode illustrates the very materials to which it testifies. It is based on the compulsive repetition of and return to the experience itself, in the absence of the ability to represent it or reflect on it. So, while the metaphoric mode of witnessing enables the shift between the first and the third persons of experience, the metonymic mode is located in the first person mode of report. This means neither that it is literally limited to the first person, nor that it is characterized by an excessive use of "I". Rather, this mode of witnessing uses no distancing, maintaining a living continuum with the traumatic memories and through it also with a sense of selfhood. The metonymic mode lacks any reflective aspect. It enacts the traumatic experience without transforming it into an integrated narrative as would be the case in the metaphoric mode, incorporating it without being capable of transcending it. In the metonymic mode of witnessing any transcendence is experienced as a split between the person and his or her identity.

To these two modes, I would like to add what I refer to as "the psychotic mode of witnessing". This mode of witnessing attacks every possible link with the trauma, separating between the person and his or her memories as well as between the person and his or her own sense of selfhood. This modality includes two sub-modalities, or two subcategories: "the *Muselmann*[5] subcategory" and "the excessive subcategory".

The *Muselmann* mode of witnessing has only rare narrative manifestations – since it essentially attacks both the ability to narrate and language itself. The post-Holocaust literature includes diverse expressions of this mode in the form of survivors' accounts, some of which appear in the form of a semi-psychotic type of discourse, both intra-psychic and inter-psychic, a discourse that annihilates any contact with the psychic reality and the pain it involves. This mode of witnessing is founded neither on the ability to shift between the first and the third person of experience (like in the metaphoric mode), nor on the capacity to stay exclusively in the first person of experience (like in the metonymic mode). In fact, it destroys both the first as well as the third person, and thereby the very possibility of an experiencing subject. This testimonial mode joins the traumatic "Real" without being able to distance itself from it on the one hand or to create a vital link with it on the other. When the dominant mode of testimony is the *Muselmann* mode – trauma turns into a "negative possession" (Amir, 2012, 2014): a psychic condition that annihilates both the capacity to represent the traumatic event as well as the ability to preserve vital contact with it.

Primo Levi (1959) writes:

> All the *Mussulmanns* who finished in the gas chambers have the same story, or more exactly, have no story; [...] the divine spark dead within them, already too empty to really suffer. One hesitates to call them living: one hesitates to call their death death, in the face of which they have no fear, as they are too tired to understand. They crowd my memory with their faceless presences, and if I could enclose all the evil of our time in one image, I would choose this image which is familiar to me: an emaciated man, with head dropped and shoulders curved, on whose face and in whose eyes not a trace of a thought is to be seen.
>
> (p. 103)

I would like to use some of Matte Blanco's ideas (Matte Blanco, 1975; Rayner, 1981) in order to try and understand how such a traumatic annihilation takes place. Matte Blanco's main claim regarding unconscious symmetric relations in primary thinking processes (such of the *Muselmann* kind), was that while most relations are "logically asymmetric", namely relations whose converses are not identical to them (for example: "a is to the *left* of b" has the converse "b is to the *right* of a") – the unconscious treats asymmetric relations as symmetric (for example: "a is to the *left* of b" will have the converse "b is to the *left* of a"). Logical thinking, which is virtually synonymous with secondary thinking processes, entertains propositions about *asymmetric* relations. *Symmetric* relations, on the other hand, are characteristic of primary thinking processes. The very conception of a whole object and its parts always presumes temporal and/or spatial asymmetric relations: if "a *includes* b" – then "b is *included* in a".

But when symmetry intervenes, the conception turns into: "a *includes* b and b *includes* a". When symmetry rules, whole objects are experienced as identical to their parts. Similarly, in ordinary logic when we discriminate that "event b *follows* event a", we will also recognise that "event a *precedes* event b". But if symmetric logic gains the upper hand – "event b *follows* event a" as well as "event a *follows* event b". When this occurs, there is no temporal sequence and time as we know it disappears (Matte Blanco, 1975; Rayner, 1981).

Laub (2014) writes similarly:

> At its core, traumatic experience is ahistorical. It does away with place and time; it happens in the here and now. Survivors may even speak in the present tense.
>
> (pp. 216–217)

Thus, since concepts of time and space do not exist in the symmetrical logic of the *Muselmann* state – the experience is that everything that happened is about to take place at any moment (Fink, 1989). This perception is a central characteristic of this mode of witnessing, which combines lack of contact with the traumatic experience along with the inability to delineate it.

A second index of primary thinking processes according to Matte Blanco is the principle of generalization. This principle is in charge of the inclusion of elements which maintain analogical relations with each other in ever more general sets or classes. In this manner, elements that are distinct in consciousness become indistinct in the unconscious due to being attributed to the same group. As a result, part and whole not only represent one another, they also become interchangeable. In effect, the further one delves into this type of thinking the more the world loses its specificity until individuals and classes finally fuse together into a "great indivisible whole" (Sanchez-Cardenas, 2011). In such conditions, which again characterize the *Muselmann* state of non-thinking – no narrative can evolve, since constituting a narrative would require a distinction between elements and an ability to respond to their singularity, along with the capacity to create movement in time and space and to establish a hierarchically based causal continuum. Amos Goldberg (2012) writes in a similar context that in the continuous trauma of their encounter with the Real, the subject is in a state of an ongoing radical invasion that erases context and blurs the differences essential for discerning and establishing identity. The breakdown of differences deprives trauma victims of their ability to create a meaningful world and thus undermines their mental stability (p. 100). LaCapra (2001) also claims that one of the dangers of trauma is the collapse of time, and along with it the distinction between internal and external as well as the distinction between the "here and now" and the "then and there". Trauma, LaCapra argues, is a "scandal" for identity and for the entire epistemological system, since it completely unravels the existing order along with its derivatives (see also Goldberg in LaCapra, 2001).

In the *Muselmann* mode, trauma operates like an impoverishing, reductive, and sterilizing mechanism, turning the entire internal discourse into one that separates both between the subject and the traumatic object as well as between the subject and his own self. In this state the subject can neither distance himself from the trauma (since it is experienced as lacking any outline in space and time – it happens now and might go on forever), nor approach it (for it is experienced as such an amorphous whole that any attempt to refer to its singularity is doomed). This form of survival is not that of the "living dead" – but rather that of the "neither dead nor alive". Erlich (1991, 2013) has formulated it as a regression to "non-being", which is the psychic expression of the death-instinct.

The excessive subcategory, by contrast, is a much more illusory one. Here the traumatic object becomes an addictive and gratifying object in its own right, one whose totality replaces the functional sense of being. In this mode of witnessing, traumatic excessiveness is available to consciousness neither by way of an elaborate link (as in the metaphoric mode) nor by way of repetition (as in the metonymic mode). Witnessing, in this case, involves the traumatic memory becoming a "saturated object" (Bion, 1959, 1962,a,b; 1970), an object that resists transformation and to which the obstinate adherence becomes malignant.

Stolorow refers to this kind of saturation in his *Trauma and Human Existence* (2007):

> When a child's perceptual and emotional experiences meet with massive and consistent invalidation, his or her belief in the reality of such experiences will remain unsteady and vulnerable to dissolution and, further, under such predisposing circumstances delusional ideas may develop that serve to dramatize and reify an endangered psychic reality ... restoring [the] vanishing belief in its validity.
>
> (p. 15)

The excessive mode of witnessing is indeed based on an extremely fragile sense of validity on the one hand, and on delusional defenses against this fragility on the other.[6] The illusiveness characteristic of this mode is related to its deceptive combination of a highly developed rhetoric on the one hand and a massive "attack on linking" (Bion, 1959) on the other. Adherence to the excessiveness of suffering and the traumatic object's imperviousness to new meanings or any other processes of change turn traumatic repetition into "a thing in itself" ("das Ding").

Lacan (1958) discusses the formation of subjectivity as being based on an experience of lack. The subject, according to him, is constituted at the point in time when he or she enters the "Symbolic order" through the mother's interpretation of the Real. Along with the experience itself, the infant is given an interpretation that renders the experience meaningful by introducing it into the order of language. Experiences that are attributed to an "identical category" come together to form what the child experiences as that category: pain, tickling, cold, missing. There is, however, always a remainder or surplus that stays outside this junction. This surplus, lost in the process of symbolization and thus remaining outside the order of language, becomes the object of desire. Psychic motion is always directed towards this object of desire and it is through this motion that the subject is constituted qua living subject. In contrast to the common concept of the satisfying object, Lacan introduces the lack of the object as constitutive to the creation of the subject in the first place. No psychic motion will ensue without the experience of lack (Amir, 2014).

The excessive mode of witnessing creates, through the consummate totality of the traumatic object, an illusion of fusion without lack, a fusion which allows a lingering in the Real at the cost of the formation of both subject and subjectivity. The deceptiveness of this mode of witnessing is related to its intensive linguistic nature: while the register of the Real precedes language and in many ways also opposes it – the overt manifestation of the excessive mode is not an absence of language. On the contrary: it often presents articulate and well-developed language, with a wealth of rhetorical features. But underneath the rhetorical surface this is a language that attacks rather than produces linking; a saturated language, one that under the guise of "full testimony" presents what Cathy Caruth (1996) calls "empty grammar": a grammar that empties the event, thus does not allow for its subjects to undergo transformation. And so, while the excessive mode might well be replete with metaphors, the metaphoric mode, as I will show, might in fact be comparatively minor and minimalistic. Rather than by the presence or absence of overt linguistic characteristics, like metaphors, these two modes are distinguished by means of whether they are employed to link or to split.

Every testimonial narrative constitutes a certain combination of these four modes, marking zones of psychic transformation versus zones of saturated thinking, zones of linking versus zones of compulsive repetition, zones in which testimony annihilates the witness versus zones in which it constitutes him or her as such.

Agamben (2002) writes:

> To bear witness is to place oneself in one's own language in the position of those who have lost it, to establish oneself in a living language as if it were dead, or in a dead language as if it were living. [...] What cannot be stated, what cannot be archived is the language in which the author succeeds in bearing witness to the incapacity to speak. In this language, a language that survives the subjects who spoke it coincides with a speaker who remains beyond it.
>
> (pp. 161–162)

Since every testimonial narrative is an intersection between "what cannot be stated" and what is actually spoken, every act of testimony is simultaneously a collapse and a formation of language: a collapse of language – since bearing witness to what cannot be testified renders testimony a meaningless event, or one that conveys "archival meaning" (Agamben, 2002) only; and a formation of language – since where language succeeds to speak not in spite of the lacuna but in its name, not beyond it but through it, it becomes a real event of testimony, one that constitutes the subject of witnessing as such.

In each of these testimonial modes language collapses in a singular way:

The metonymic mode collapses into repetition, allowing no room for reflection. It creates an experiential continuity between subject and traumatic event, thereby preserving a psychic outline, but in fact remains trapped in this outline without the freedom to retrospectively reconstruct the traumatic memory.

The excessive mode collapses into rhetoric. Via linguistic excessiveness, it creates an artificial bridge over the traumatic lacuna, but this excessiveness does not create a vital link: it rather constitutes a hollow, addictive syntax which fixates the traumatic object at the center while pushing the reflective subject to the margins.

The *Muselmann* mode collapses into the traumatic abyss itself. Here is where testimony is at its fullest and emptiest simultaneously: one that is present only in the form of its absence.

The metaphoric mode collapses into language while also constituting language. To this Agamben alludes when he speaks of the ability to intersect what is said with what cannot be stated: the *Muselmann* with the survivor. This is the only mode that can contain the uncanny "background noise", which cannot be transformed, along with the "speaker who remains beyond it" (Agamben, p. 162). The movement between different states (the position of the victim and the position of the witness, the experiential I and the narrating I, the familiar and the uncanny) which the metaphoric mode enables, creates the necessary intersection of dead language with living language. Amos Goldberg (2012) writes that "trauma is directed opposite to the trajectory of a life story" (p. 102). One can therefore think of the metaphoric mode as the site of struggle between the formative power of the life story and the destructive power of the trauma, with the latter prevailing.

Dominick LaCapra (1994, 2001) argues that texts about the Holocaust show two forms of cultural and political coping with trauma. Following Freud, he refers to one as a type of "acting out" and to the other as "working through". The first is characterized by an unconscious repetition of post-traumatic symptoms, while the other involves the critical control of the trauma, with the aim of counteracting the compulsive repetition. LaCapra further identifies two forms of writing that belong to the "acting out" category: The first is the "fetish" aim to deny the fundamental undermining created by trauma. It is an attempt to impose conservative and closed conventions, which generate a redemptive narrative maintaining the pretension of understanding the historic events and of granting them meaning in a way that redeems them from their incomprehensibility (Goldberg, introduction to LaCapra, 2006, Hebrew edition). Another type of acting out is expressed in post-structural writing about the Holocaust, which reenacts basic aspects of the traumatic experience itself (ibid.). LaCapra identifies this style as a cultural post-traumatic syndrome in which the past returns through the text's stylistic features.

Against these two poetics of acting out, LaCapra posits a poetics of working-through, which invokes processes of mourning. Referring to

Laplanche and Pontalis he argues that "working through would thus seem to involve a mode of repetition, offering a measure of critical purchase on problems and responsible control in action which would permit desirable change" (LaCapra, 1994, p. 209). Working-through, according to LaCapra, neither denies the excessive and boundary breaching aspects of trauma nor becomes addicted to trauma's un-availability to representation and knowledge. This is an attempt to find the balance between full control and total fragmentation; between fixed identity and the illusive, threatening, disruptive dimension of dealing with trauma.

One might draw a parallel between LaCapra's two forms of acting out and the excessive, metonymic and Muselmann modes presented here: the excessive mode constitutes the traumatic object as "saturated" and hermetic, thus attaining alleged control at the expense of the ability to be in touch with trauma's destructive qualities. This is similar to LaCapra's fetishistic style and suffers from similar disadvantages. His post-structural style, on the other hand, shares some of the characteristics of the metonymic mode (which preserves the link with the trauma through the reenactment of its characteristics) and the *Muselmann* mode (which preserves contact with the traumatic lacuna by becoming a lacuna itself). The poetics of working-through, by contrast, somewhat resembles what I referred to as the metaphoric mode, which attains a balance between the controlling and the fragmenting aspects, or between safeguarding the narrator and surrendering to the narrative.

The next chapters will discuss various literary as well as raw testimonies in an attempt to trace the way in which these four modes of witnessing interact in every single testimonial narrative, ranging along an entire span of malignant and benign relations with the traumatic object.

Notes

1 *Ces Parents Qui Vivent A Travers Moi.*

2 Gerson (2009) refers to this as "the dead third": "The 'dead third' is conceptualized as the loss of a 'live third' upon whom the individual had previously relied, had entrusted with faith, and in relation to whom or which, had developed a sense of personal continuity and meaning. In this regard, the third [...] serves the elemental function of solidifying an individual's sense of person, place, and purpose. [...] Under such circumstances, the living thirds in which the person was nested now become a nest of dead thirds from which he or she cannot escape" (ibid., p. 1343).

3 The link between trauma and the unleashing of the death instinct derivatives can be found in Freud's reference to the negative effects of trauma leading to "an inhibition – even an inability to deal with life" (Freud, quoted in Kirshner, 1994, p. 238).

4 I draw on Astrid Erll (2011b, see also 2011a in this context) for whom "the distinction between an 'experiencing I' and a 'narrating I' already rests on a (largely implicit) concept of memory", or in other words, on the idea that there is a difference between pre-narrative experience on the one hand, and, on the other, narrative memory which creates meaning retrospectively.

5 *Muselmann* (*pl. Muselmänner*, German for Muslim) was a term used among captives of Nazi concentration camps to refer to those of their fellow captives who, suffering from a combination of starvation (known also as "hunger disease") and exhaustion, had become apathetically resigned to their impending death.

6 Stolorow's definition of "delusional", following Atwood, is "ideas whose validity is not open for discussion" (p. 15). If we refer to "discussion" as a representation of an external as well as internal dialogue – "not open for discussion" may in fact be understood as "not open for any kind of transformation".

References

Agamben, G. (2002). *Remnants of Auschwitz: The witness and the archive*. (trans: D. Heller-Roazen). New York: Zone Books.

Amir, D. (2012). The inner witness. *International Journal of Psycho-Analysis*, 93, 879–896.

Amir, D. (2014). *Cleft tongue: The language of psychic structures*. London: Karnac Books.

Amir, D. (2015). From the narrative of the victim to the narrative of the witness: Traumatic testimony. *Journal of Literature and Trauma Studies*, 3(1), 43–62.

Amir, D. (2016). When language meets the traumatic lacuna: The metaphoric, the metonymic and the psychotic modes of testimony. *Psychoanalytic Inquiry* 36(8), 620–632.

Bion, W. (1959). Attacks on linking. *International Journal of Psycho-Analysis*, 40, 308–315.

Bion, W. (1962a). *Learning from experience*. New York: Basic Books.

Bion, W. (1962b). The psycho-analytic study of thinking. *International Journal of Psycho-Analysis*, 43, 306–310.

Bion, W. (1970). *Attention and interpretation*. London: Tavistock.

Camus, A. ([1956] 2004). *The plague, the fall, exile and the kingdom, and selected essays*. (trans. Justin O'Brien). New York: Everyman's Library.

Camus, A. ([1956] 2004). The fall (La Chute). In: A. Camus, *The plague, the fall, exile and the kingdom, and selected essays*. (trans. J. O'Brien). New York: Everyman's Library .

Caruth, C. (1996). *Unclaimed experience: Trauma narrative and history*. Baltimore, MD: Johns Hopkins University Press.

Erlich, H. S. (1991). "Being" and "doing" in psychoanalysis and psychotherapy. *Zeitschrift fuer psychoanalytische Theorie und Praxis [Journal for Psychoanalytic Theory and Practice]*, 6, 317–334.

Erlich, H. S. (2013). "Whose trauma is it?" A lecture given in the Israel Psychoanalytic Society, 5 November, Jerusalem.

Erll, A. (2011a). *Memory in culture*. Basingstoke, UK: Palgrave Macmillan.

Erll, A. (2011b). Travelling memory. *Parallax, Special Issue: Transcultural Memory*, 17(4), 4–18.
Felman, S. (1992). Camus' the plague, or a monument to witnessing. In: S. Felman and D. Laub (Eds.), *Testimony: Crises of witnessing in literature, psychoanalysis, and history* (pp. 93–119). New York: Routledge.
Fink, K. (1989). From symmetry to asymmetry. *International Journal of Psycho-Analysis*, 70, 481–489.
Gampel, Y. (1999). Between the background of safety and the background of uncanny in the context of social violence. In: E. Bott Spillius (Editor in Chief), *Psychoanalysis on the move*, (pp. 59–74). London: Routledge.
Gampel, Y. (2010). *Ces Parents Qui Vivent A Travers Moi* [*The parents who live through me*], (trans: T. Mishor). Jerusalem: Keter.
Gampel, Y. and Mazor, A. (2004). Intimacy and family links of adults who were children during the Shoa: Multi-faceted mutations of the traumatic encapsulations. *Free Associations*, 11(4), 556–568.
Gerson, S. (2009). When the third is dead: Memory, mourning, and witnessing in the aftermath of the Holocaust. *International Journal of Psycho-Analysis*, 90, 1341–1357.
Goldberg, A. (2006). Introduction. In: LaCapra, D. (Ed.), *Writing history, writing trauma*. (trans: Y. Farkash). Tel Aviv, Israel: Riesling.
Goldberg, A. (2007). "The era of the witness". A lecture given at the Scholion Centre, the Hebrew University, 1 January, Jerusalem.
Goldberg, A. (2012). *Trauma in first person*. Or Yehuda, Israel: Kinneret, Zmora-Bitan, Dvir Publishing House; Beer-Sheva, Israel: Heksherim Institute, Ben Gurion University of the Negev.
Jakobson, R. (1956). Two aspects of language and two types of aphasic disturbances. In: Jacobson, R. (1971) (Ed.), *Selected writings – word and language volume 2* (pp. 239–259). Den-Haag, Paris: Mouton.
Kirshner, L. A. (1994). Trauma, the good object, and the symbolic: A theoretical integration. *International Journal of Psycho-Analysis*, 75, 235–242.
Kohut, H. (1971). *The analysis of the self.* New York: International Universities Press.
Lacan, J. ([1958] 2007). *Écrits*. (trans: B. Fink). London: W. W. Norton.
Lacan, J. (1977). The function and field of speech and language in psychoanalysis. In: *Ecrits* ([1958] 2007) (pp. 30–113). (trans: A. Sheridan). New York: Norton.
LaCapra, D. (1994). *Representing the Holocaust: History, theory, trauma*. New York: Cornell University.
LaCapra, D. (2001). *Writing history, writing trauma*. Baltimore, MD: Johns Hopkins University Press.
Laub, D. (2005). Traumatic shutdown of narrative and symbolization. *Contemporary Psychoanalysis*, 41, 307–326.
Laub, D. (2014). Scholar's Forum Engaging survivors: Assessing 'testimony' and 'trauma' as foundational concepts. *Dapim: Studies on the Holocaust*, 28(3), 190–226.

Laub, D. and Auerhahn, N. (1993). Knowing and not knowing: Forms of traumatic memory. *International Journal of Psycho-Analysis*, 74, 287–302.

Levi, P. ([1958] 1959). *If this is a man*. (trans: S. Woolf). New York: The Orion Press.

Liska, V. (2009). After the silence: Holocaust remembrance in contemporary Austrian-Jewish literature. In: *When Kafka says we: Uncommon communities in German-Jewish literature* (pp. 151–159). Bloomington and Indianapolis: Indiana University Press.

Matte Blanco, I. (1975). *The unconscious as infinite sets. An essay in bi-logic*. London: Gerald Duckworth & Company Limited.

Modell, A. (2006). *Imagination and the meaningful brain*. Cambridge, MA: MIT Press.

Moore, R. (1999). *The creation of reality in psychoanalysis*. Hillsdale, NJ: The Analytic Press.

Oliner, M. (1996). External reality: The elusive dimensions of psychoanalysis. *Psychoanalytic Quarterly*, 65, 267–300.

Rayner E. (1981). Infinite experiences, affects and the characteristics of the unconscious. *International Journal of Psycho-Analysis*, 62, 403–412.

Sanchez-Cardenas, M. (2011). Matte Blanco's thought and epistemological pluralism in psychoanalysis. *International Journal Psycho-Analysis*, 92, 811–831.

Stern, D. B. (2012). Witnessing across time: Accessing the present from the past and the past from the present. *Psychoanalytic Quarterly*, 81, 53–81.

Stolorow, R. D. (2007). *Trauma and human existence: Autobiographical, psychoanalytic, and philosophical reflections*. New York: Routledge.

Van der Kolk, B., McFarlane, A. and Weisaeth, L. (1996). *Traumatic stress: The effects of overwhelming experience on mind, body, and society*. New York: The Guilford Press.

Chapter 2

Autobiographical fiction or fictional autobiography?

Georges Perec's *W, or the Memory of Childhood*[1]

Georges Perec's book *W, or the Memory of Childhood* (2010 [1975]) consists of two seemingly unrelated texts that are nevertheless intricately and thus inseparably intertwined. While one is a fictional text, and the other presumes to be an autobiographical account, neither is entirely what it claims to be. The fictional clearly carries autobiographical elements, while the autobiographical often straddles the boundary between reality and fiction.

The narrator presents his "witness position" quite at the beginning of this book: "I am not the hero of my tale", he proclaims, "Nor am I exactly its bard" (p. 4). Not only was he a passive eye witness rather than an agent in relation to the past events, as a present witness, too, he tells a story that is not his.

We may indeed describe the movement between the different modes of testimony in terms of degrees of ownership: in the metaphoric mode of testimony, the witness is both owner and hero of his or her story. Even if he or she narrates it from a completely passive point of view, the text is experienced as belonging to them. In the metonymic mode, on the other hand, the witness is led by the story rather than the latter being led by the witness, whereas in the psychotic mode, neither story nor witness lead: instead, there is a standstill caused by the disappearance of reference points, leading to total disorientation. This standstill can manifest itself as an excessiveness that obstructs any movement to and from the "frozen" original story, or alternatively as an attack on the entire thinking apparatus which undermines any possibility of creating a meaningful story, not to mention the possibility of owning it.

Thus, by emphasizing "I am not the hero of my tale. Nor am I exactly its bard" (p. 4), the narrator touches on the question of his relation to the traumatic events to which he bears witness. This question, concerning the possibility of being the owner of his own biography, will be discussed throughout his book in many complex variations.

The narrator's first attempt to engage the above question is through the presentation of two biographical statements at the beginning of the book:

The first statement (which appears in Chapter 1) recounts his father's death when the narrator was 6 years old; the narrator's subsequent adoption by a neighbor who raised him as a workman; his enlistment in the army, his desertion with the help of an organization of conscientious objectors, his subsequent move to Germany, finding a job as a garage mechanic and spending most of his evenings at a bar. In this biographical statement, his mother is not mentioned. The second biographical statement (in Chapter 2) begins with the words: "I have no childhood memories", immediately followed by an alternative biography which, while interacting with some aspects of the first one, completely differs from it. In this biographical variant, his father died when he was 4 and his mother died when he was 6; he resided in various boarding schools during the war and was eventually adopted by his father's sister and her husband.

The setting up of two biographical variants, one alongside the other, conveys a message that cuts across this entire testimonial text: where there is no "continuous core" (Amir, 2016), what we call "biography" is no more than the singular way in which the narrator "fills in" the empty holes and blind spots of memory with his unconscious projections and phantasies. This is why different variants can certainly exist for the same biography. As we will see further on, the narrator interweaves "living" memories, which he refutes no sooner than he has recounted them, with "dead" memories that did in fact occur – but to which he has no vital link. That these two types of memory keep occurring, side by side, is no coincidence. It reflects the author's determination not to choose between them.

As we progress through the allegedly autobiographical and the fictional parts alike, it becomes clear that even the memories the narrator has "borrowed" from others, as he declares, are not random. In certain cases, it seems that the only way for him to preserve a vital link with his nameless pains is by means of "borrowing" from other's biography "plots" that can make those pains meaningful, and in that way deposit them within himself.

One example is a dubious memory of an event that turned out to not have happened at all: the memory is of his scapula being broken after he crashed into a sled while skating. As a result of this fracture, his right arm was "strapped" behind his back to allow the scapula to heal. Further on, he tells of an encounter in 1970 with a friend who told him that the accident, which he clearly remembered, did not happen to him but to another friend. He most likely witnessed it, but was certainly not its victim:

> I can see perfectly well what it was that these easily mendable fractures, which could be remedied simply by keeping them still for a stretch, were meant to stand in for, although today it seems to me that the metaphor will not serve as a way of describing what had been broken – and what it was surely pointless hoping to contain within the guise of an imaginary limb.
>
> (p. 80)

Thus, these fractures which he invented as memories, these "marks of suspension", as he names them, "indicated pains that could be named" (p. 80) and thereby served to justify his need for attention, the real cause of which remained unspoken. But beyond their undeniable symbolic significance, one can view these planted, fictitious memories, as another attempt to construct his life as a continuous story. Since the pain he felt was psychical and not physical, and since the psychical pain remained unspoken, the only way to explain this pain to himself was to make up physical injuries that would serve as a reason. The tales of fractures and injuries were part of this child's attempt to establish a coherent sequence, to rehabilitate the thinking apparatus which was under constant attack by the arbitrariness of the experienced reality and which lacked the discursive access that could endow it with meaning (Amir, 2017). This was achieved by creating a story that could render those experiences meaning in terms of causality (I was injured and therefore I'm in pain), space (I was injured as a result of crashing into a sledge while ice-skating) and time (the crash preceded the pain which preceded the binding of the scapula). It was his way of defending his incessantly attacked thinking apparatus by creating "a-symmetrical" relations where "symmetric logic" (Matte Blanco, 1975) hitherto prevailed.

Since the narrator lacks the experience of being either hero or owner of his story – writing turns into an act of weaving, placing biographical and allegedly biographical strips across one another in order to create the fabric of memory. The narrator demands that the reader will be an active witness – in contrast to the passive witness he himself chooses to be – so as to create, on behalf of him, an act of integration. Just as he borrows the memories of others, so he borrows the reader's ability to connect, in order to stitch together what he himself cannot make into one piece.

> I was excused [from the question about the nature of his history, D.A.]: a different history, History with a capital H, had answered the question in my stead: the war, the camps.
>
> (p. 6)

One of the most difficult tasks in bearing witness to trauma is, indeed, that of discerning between personal and general history. It is so easy, the narrator suggests, to use the objective history in order to erase the subjective one; so easy to use *history* to erase *biography*. When the inner witness (Amir, 2012) is fragile and unstable, History with a capital H offers a means of escape, holding out articulation and expression, and providing an artificial coating and context.

When he was 13 years old, the narrator recalls, he wrote and illustrated the story W, which constitutes the book's main fictional part. This situates W, the fictional story parallel to the autobiographical one within the narrator's own autobiography ("if not the story of my childhood, then at least a story of my childhood" – p. 6), mixing up again the allegedly biographical and the allegedly fictional parts of the book:

> W is no more like my Olympic fantasy than that Olympic fantasy was like my childhood. But in the crisscross web they weave as in my reading of them I know there is to be found the inscription and the description of the path I have taken, the passage of my history and the story of my passage.
>
> (p. 7)

Testimony is not just "the story of the passage", but also "the passage of the story": rather than a two-dimensional text that lists the facts, it weaves and revives these facts, often precisely through memory's tortuous paths and mazes. In this sense, the story of the passage, that is, the manner in which the story is both internalized and externalized, is no less important than the passage of the story.

> For years I had tried to sidetrack or to cover up these obvious facts, and I wrapped myself in the harmless status of the orphan, the unparented,

> the nobody's boy. However, childhood is neither longing nor terror, neither a paradise lost nor the Golden Fleece, but maybe it is a horizon, a point of departure, a set of coordinates from which the axes of my life may draw their meaning. [...] I have no alternative but to conjure up what for too many years I called the irrevocable: the things that were, the things that stopped, the things that were closed off – things that surely were and today are no longer, but things that also were so that I may still be.
>
> (pp. 12–13)

Where childhood is either terror or a Golden Fleece, the nostalgic lost paradise – the ability to bear witness is obliterated: these are the areas where the position of the witness is lost, since the psyche, overwhelmed by either idealization or anxiety, cannot hold on to the story. Thus, as he goes back to his childhood, he refutes each memory no sooner than he recalls it, turns it upside down, strips it of one meaning and attributes another, presenting the recollection as part hallucination, part fantasy and part dream.

The first memory he mentions is an excellent example: he is three years old, he says, and all the members of his family have gathered around the baby "which was just born" (a moment later he wonders, in parenthesis: "but didn't I say a moment ago that I was three?" – p. 13). The spectators are in awe since the baby has just pointed to a Hebrew letter and called it by its name. He remembers identifying the letter "ג" ('gimmel'), yet the letter he remembers looks nothing like a Hebrew gimmel, rather resembling a gaping, upside down variation of the Hebrew character "mem" ("מ"). In addition, the painting which the recollection reminds him of ("Jesus amid the Doctors") doesn't actually feature Jesus the infant, as one might expect, but rather the adult Jesus. This memory is so unreliable that it undermines not only itself but any possibility of memory. The letter is not the letter, the painting is not the painting, the infant's age is not his age, and further on the narrator recounts having been told that he knew how to recognize French letters but certainly not Hebrew letters – thus could not have recognized the Hebrew letter as he allegedly did in his recollection.

The significance of this detailed scrutiny of his childhood memory is not necessarily related to the particular memory itself – but to the way in which it disintegrates in the attempt to grasp it. It's as if the narrator wants to prove both to himself and the reader, as he does many times throughout this book, that there is no such thing as a childhood memory.

Since memory is a fiction fabricated through deferred action, it resembles a dream narrative much more than any form of historic documentation.

The second memory the narrator introduces has several versions that keep changing and tipping over:

> The simplest statement of it would be this: my father comes home from his work; he gives me a key. In one version, the key is made of gold. In another version it is not a golden key, but a gold coin; in yet another version, I am on the potty when my father comes home from his work; and, finally, in yet another version, I swallow the coin, everyone fusses, and the next day it turns up in my stool.
>
> (pp. 13–14)

Here, too, the description comes to bear out the built-in illusion of memory. As we move back and forth between the different versions, we try to find something to keep hold of in order to determine whether it was a key or a coin, whether he received it, swallowed it and then excreted it, or just received it, or perhaps never received it at all. What appears consistent throughout the versions is that the father returns home from work and that there is a boy who awaits him; the latter receives something from the former or perhaps expects something of him, yearns for him but may also be angry at him (since he swallows the coin but also excretes it, thus turning the golden key/coin into feces).

This thin thread of the child's expectation from his father, and perhaps also his yearning to grant him a gift in return (in the only productive way he knows, which is by defecating) – can indeed be detected in the various versions. What seems important is that this thread only becomes manifest when one examines the combination of all versions while cannot be observed in any single one of them alone. Apparently, it is the abundance of factual and fictitious variations that brings to the fore what repeats itself and therefore proves important: a father, a child, a gift that is swallowed and ejected.

This relation between essential and incidental, or between the factual and the fictitious, has a constant symbolic presence in this book through the relations between the main text and the footnotes: throughout, the footnotes appear in a similar font as the main text and as its continuation. Not only are they not "footnotes" in terms of their length and content, but the text itself is often situated as a reference to them. This blurring between center and margins, between essential and incidental, is the very issue Perec addresses in this book with regard to the subject of testimony: What is essential and what is incidental? Does truth reside in the facts or in our unconscious phantasies?

This question resonates in the story of Jasper Winkler, the boy after whom the narrator of the first fictitious part of the book is called. Jasper Winkler was a sickly and puny, deaf and dumb eight-year-old son of a famous Austrian singer who found refuge in Switzerland during the war. In order to alleviate his suffering and in the hope of curing his infirmity, which was diagnosed as psychosomatic rather than organic, his mother took him on a trip around the world. Due to a technical error, the narrator was given the boy's passport, enabling his own escape, while the child was listed in his mother's passport. The boy and his mother set out on their expedition: As the days went by, hopes of the boy's recovery diminished, turning the trip into an erratic wandering in futile search for a place "where suddenly it could all happen – the veil sundered, the light turned on" (p. 24).

One day, a cyclone hit the ship on which mother and son were traveling and it sank. Upon reaching the ship, the rescue team found five corpses, which did not include the boy's body. Otto Apfelstahl, who traced Winkler (the protagonist) in order to ask for his help in solving this mystery – asks him to set out on an expedition to find his lost double, the boy with the same name. Otto has been able to trace the circumstances of the shipwreck and has concluded that it is unlikely that the boy fell off the board. There is, hence, a possibility that the boy escaped the ship at some earlier stage, and that the ship turned back to look for him. Another possibility is that they abandoned him and only later regretted it and returned.

What is the significance of connecting this first fictitious story, which breaks off in the middle and has no continuation whatsoever, with the second fictitious story in this book – the tale of the fictional island of W? And what is the relationship between each of these stories and the story of the narrator's own childhood?

The story of Jasper Winkler is probably the book's most mysterious part, mostly since it opens up something that will never be resolved. The five chapters revolving around the fate of Jasper Winkler are written like a suspense story. The reader's expectation from this genre is that the mysterious details eventually add up to one, fairly tight plot. Here, however, the exact opposite happens. The details don't add up at all, and if, for a moment, they seem to merge and form some kind of pointer – we discover all too soon that this is a false track. These chapters' resemblance to a detective story is an illusion, a signpost leading to a dead-end, thus constituting one more enactment of the theme that Perec repeats in this book in every possible variation: his biography is a path leading to no horizon that he can identify.

Perec himself relates to this in his introductory note:

> [...] the adventure story is rather grandiose, or maybe dubious. For it begins to tell one tale, and then, all of a sudden, launches into another. In this break, in this split suspending the story on an unidentifiable expectation, can be found the point of departure for the whole of this book.

Thus, the content here is enacted by the form, creating in the reader's experience a reconstruction of the writer's detached and aimless stance.

It is not difficult, however, to see the similarities between Jasper Winkler's story of disappearance and the story of Perec's own childhood. Both stories feature a boy who sets out on a journey which is supposed to save him from his deafness and dumbness. While the first boy's deafness and dumbness are presented as concrete phenomena (though it is implied that they have no organic cause and may rather be post-traumatic), the second boy suffers from a deafness and dumbness in relation to his childhood memories. While the disappearance of one child is a concrete one – the other, unable to trace his own biography, disappears symbolically.

Both stories recount an experience of fragmentation. In both cases, the story does not unfold along a distinct chronological and causal continuum. They both feature a traumatic event (one or more) that tears a rift in the story, alongside an attempt to mend this rift: the narrator does this by means of writing his memoirs, and Winkler by setting out in a symbolic search of his missing double. In both stories, abandonment and rescue intermingle: the deaf boy is taken on a rescue journey during which he is most probably abandoned, while Perec the child is sent on a journey, which he experiences as his mother's abandonment of him, in order to be saved. The letter W that connects all three stories (the autobiographic[2] and the two fictional ones) indicates that horror weaves through all three of them like an invisible thread and that this perplexity is their common subject. W signifies the lacuna. The place where memory collapses into fiction, but no less the place where fiction collapses into memory.

In the allegedly autobiographical chapters of the book, the narrator recounts how he "made up" the image of his father, who died "a slow and stupid death" (p. 29), reinventing him as a figure who died heroically. Similarly, he makes up his mother's history, by way of a compilation of Andersen's *The Little Match Girl* and Cosette from *Les Miserables*, weaving in biographical descriptions which he constantly contradicts in the footnotes. As suggested before, the narrator inserts struggle and unease between text and footnotes. He contrives this by means of the sheer length and location of the footnotes as well as through their clashing content, thus creating a circular experience of construction, fragmentation and reconstruction. In that way he reconstructs his mother's history but maintains the fictitious version by its side, omitting to arbitrate between them. There is no "correction" in light of the facts: instead, concrete facts and fiction blend into a single fabric in which incoherency is the main rule.

It is no coincidence that in describing his mother's life, future and past get mixed up so that here he seems not to allow her to grow up while elsewhere he makes her older than she really was. As the time of trauma is circular, he can place her anywhere in time or even outside time. But due to this same circularity he feels again and again cast outside any possible continuity, in a way that prevents him, too, from generating a hierarchy of any sort (time and space, cause and effect, essential and incidental). Since he does not own the story he tells, the narrating subject himself becomes in this text a sort of illusion. Perhaps this explains the sudden shift to the third person when he describes a photograph of himself and his mother:[3] "mother and child make a picture of happiness" (p. 49). Interestingly, this movement into a more remote, impersonal mode of description occurs when he points to an experience rather than when he deals with facts (he describes details of dress and facial features, for instance, in the first person). It is the experience, not the facts, that he does not own.

In the same chapter, he describes another photograph in which he appears by his mother's side in a Parisian park. Here, too, he renders in minute detail his and her attire, her facial features as well as his own face. On the edge of the photo one may glimpse something that could be part of the overcoat of the person taking the picture, who might be his father; and in the background appears a little girl in a light-colored coat. These two details, supposedly marginal, shed light on the portrait to which this picture is really dedicated: the portrait of the absent, of what the picture cannot contain: a dead father and a little sister who didn't survive after her birth. It is no coincidence that he recounts that his first memories pertain to the period after the escape from Paris and not before it and that he has no recollection of the flight itself (p. 51): the flight, much like the figures of the dead father and the still-born sister, was a missed traumatic event, remaining outside the frame of his memory picture.

Three anecdotes are registered in his memory from his days at school (p. 53).[4] Of these three memories, the first is the haziest: they are crowded in the school basement, trying on their gas masks. He recalls big eyes (probably the goggles that are part of the mask), a protruding object dangling from the front and a nauseating smell of rubber. In this recollection, there is reference neither to fear nor to the reason for trying on these masks. Thus, it is only in mentioning the nausea and the image of the "big eyes" that his anxiety, neither spoken nor experienced at the time, is somehow reflected.

The second memory describes him as a boy rushing down the street, holding a colorful drawing of a brown bear on a dark brown background, and calling out *here come the cubs, here come the cubs*. A seemingly innocent, even joyful childhood memory. Yet, here, too, context is lacking. It is unclear either what the boy is running from, or indeed where to; it is also unclear whether somebody sent him or is waiting for him. The unknown that lurks in the center of this memory picture constitute, as it were, the boy's addressee: the figure towards which he directs his movement in space.

The third recollection is the most coherent one. Here he receives a medal for good behavior at school, and the medal is pinned to his smock. He is halfway up the staircase, which is crowded at the end of the school day, when someone shoves him and falls on top of him, thus making him accidentally push a little girl standing by his side. The teacher pounces on him and tears the medal from his smock. He remembers himself running down the street, and the sense of that shove in his back, which caused him to lose his balance, is so powerfully imprinted on his memory that he wonders whether it conceals its opposite: "not the memory of a star torn off, but the memory of a star pinned on" (p. 54).

Whether this memory does or does not conceal the memory of the yellow star (which as we later learn is a collective memory rather than a personal one, for the narrator himself was never required to wear the yellow star), the sense of injustice and arbitrariness, the sudden whimsical change from good to bad, the reversal of the caressing hand into the hand that strikes – all this cuts across his entire childhood experience.

The relation between memory and reality resembles here the relation between conscious thinking and dream: the memory, just like the dream, is saturated with symbolic distortions, relations that are difficult to comprehend, facts that masquerade as other facts (a yellow star of David poses as a medal), all that in order to protect the psyche from an unbearable encounter with painful contents while at the same time enabling that encounter.

The fourth memory, which not by chance emerged while writing, is of a childhood pastime in which he would place colorful cardboard strips cross-wise over each other, so as to form paper placemats. It seems that contrary to reality's guiding rules which were almost impossible to discern, in this simple game the guiding principle was apparent and clear. Contrary to the disrupted sense of continuity – how immense was the binding power of weaving.

> What marks this period especially is the absence of landmarks: these memories are scraps of life snatched from the void. No mooring. Nothing to anchor them or hold them down. Almost no way of ratifying them. No sequence in time, except as I have reconstructed it arbitrarily over the years [...].
>
> (pp. 68–69)

The chronology – if there is any to speak of – is arbitrary: the product of a reconstruction based on a random and meaningless choice of details which do not form a real continuum:

> No beginning, no end. There was no past, and for very many years there was no future either; things simply went on. You were there. It happened somewhere far away, but no one could have said very precisely where it was far from [...]. Things and places had no name, or several; the people had no faces. One time it was an aunt, next time it was another aunt. Or a grandmother. [...] You didn't ask for anything, you didn't really know what you should ask for, you must have been a bit afraid of the answer you'd get if you did make up your mind to ask for something. You didn't ask any questions. You waited for fate to bring auntie back, or if not that aunt, then the other – in the end you didn't much care which one it was and anyway you didn't really care whether there were any aunties at all or not. [...] You could get by in life quite well without, you couldn't really see the point, nor why these

> people were more important than the others [...]. The only thing you do know is that it went on for years and then one day it stopped.
>
> (p. 69)

This text precisely describes the thinking processes characteristic of the *Muselmann*-mode of testimony: the absence of a sense of space (it is unclear what the distance is and between which two points it extends), the absence of a sense of time ("The only thing you do know is that it went on for years and then one day it stopped"), the absence of a sense of specificity resulting in an inability to discriminate one object from another ("In the end you didn't much care which one it was and anyway you didn't really care whether there were any aunties at all or not"). In the territory of symmetrical logic, as suggested by Matte Blanco (1975), objects undergo ongoing generalization until they become an indiscriminate bloc. The ability to remember the past – like the ability to imagine the future – implies the ability to diverge from the present. When there is no experience of time and space, it is hence impossible to stray from the concrete present, whether forwards, backwards or inwards.

In an attempt to mend the cracks in his thinking, Perec reads books, trying to internalize their sequential plots:

> [...] not only as if I had always known them but, much more, as if they were, to my mind, virtually part of history: an inexhaustible fount of memory, of material for rumination and of a kind of certainty: the words were where they should be, and the books told a story you could follow; you could re-read, and on re-reading, re-encounter, enhanced by the certainty that you would encounter those words again, the impression you had felt the first time.
>
> (pp. 142–143)

The books provided what life took away: a sense of linearity, of narrative continuity. For in these books the words remained, images and episodes stayed fixed in their places, the plot proceeded sequentially and logically; there was a beginning and an end instead of a merely circular, senseless movement. Literature, as opposed to life, provided conditions that enabled the rehabilitation of thinking.

What was striking about the first three books that captivated him, was that they were "incomplete books": either they had a sequel which he didn't know or a beginning he hadn't read: "they presupposed other absent and unfindable books" (p. 143). So, on the one hand, those books created a stable reality which provided conditions for thinking, but on the other hand they, too, concealed black holes, blind spots, lacunae of all sorts. They simultaneously rehabilitated the reality of his childhood but also repeated it, preserving contact with it by virtue of the fact that they too, like him, lacked something that preceded or followed them.

Although in terms of the described content, this traumatic zone creates a psychotic mode of experience – Perec's testimonial mode in *The Memory of Childhood* chapters is not psychotic, but rather a metonymic one which enacts in the reader's experience the thing to which it testifies: feelings of disintegration and lack of orientation, as well as an experience of being "external" to the narrative sequence. This external experience is enacted by means not only of the content, but also through the detachment of the autobiographical part from the fictional part in a way that makes it very difficult to put them together in terms of any continuity. Thus, despite its rich symbolic language, Perec's autobiographical writing is one in which by means of metonymy a psychotic experience is transferred. Often the content meets the criteria characterizing the psychotic mode (which resists both thinking and memory), while the form (fragmented and non-cumulative) metonymically enacts this content in the reader's response.

Much more misleading in its allegorical richness – Perec's fictional writing meets the criteria of a psychotic excessive testimonial mode. Contrary to the autobiographical text, the fictional story of *the island of W* is tightly knit, has a clear narrative sequence, laden with details that follow a calculated and exact logic, without associative deviations or slippages into the inner world of the narrator. However, this excessively rigid and detached text forms a distinctly testimonial narrative in itself. For the text not only suffers from all the characteristics of the regime of *the Island of W*, but also enacts them on the reader who find themselves lost in the abundance of details, collapsing under the burden of the laws and their implications, trapped helpless in the logic of the horror which gradually strangles his or her own capacity to remember and think.

Perec's authorial position in the story of W, even more than in any of the chapters of *The Memory of Childhood* includes no narrating I that is capable of bearing witness to himself. As such, through a process that resembles projective identification, it deposits in the reader the demand not only to bear witness to the actual contents – but also to struggle against the "attack on thinking" caused by the absence of a narrating I. The excessive-psychotic quality of this testimonial text, thus, is not manifested in the rhetorical abundance, full of pathos, described above as the main characteristic of the excessive testimonial mode – but rather originates in the suffocating, hermetic wealth of details that flood the reader and finally block his or her inner ability to autonomously react to them. Despite being a story – the W chapters include no plot. On the contrary: they constitute an obsessively dry report which does not miss any technical detail – but which at the same time persistently passes over any detail that might create a specific image or character. Instead of a story told from the specific perspective of one narrator, conveying through the private laboratory of his personality and history the story of the state as a whole – the story of W is recounted in an encyclopedic style without any personal point of view, opinion or experience.

There seems to be a fundamental contradiction between the lack of hierarchy and logic that typifies (and nullifies) the chapters of *The Memory of Childhood* and the rigid organizing principle of the W chapters, as if these are two clashing territories of thinking: the one is characterized by a symmetrical logic in which the rules blend into one another so relentlessly that they result in an experience of no rules, an experience in which nothing follows and is discriminated from anything; whereas the other is enacted by an absolutely a-symmetrical logic, in which rules and regulations cover every area of thinking and nothing is left to imagination or arbitrariness.

In the course of reading, however, it appears that what was set up as a contradiction is in fact one and the same thing, for both territories are crucially marked by the absence of a narrating I: Whether it sinks into the abyss of non-memory, or it is worn down under the oppressive wheels of the encyclopedic memory – it is equally absent in both. Not surprisingly, towards the end of the book, the W child and Perec are linked: "a W child knows almost nothing of the world in which he will live" (p. 137).

Perec writes in the preface:

> In this break [...] can be found the point of departure for the whole of this book: the *points of suspension* on which the broken threads of childhood and the web of writing are caught.

While seemingly aiming to create a sort of puzzle which strives to connect its different pieces – the connection never happens. W does not connect to

"The Memory of Childhood"; It remains unclear how Winkler and W are related; there are indications of a suspense story or a mystery crime – but what happens is the very opposite: while the parts of a regular suspense story are eventually woven together into a conclusion that sheds light on everything, including that which seemed marginal and incidental – here the parts not only fail to intertwine, but rather continue to fall apart. This story ends as it begins, with no attempt to clearly demarcate its margins or mark its center. *W, or the Memory of Childhood* chillingly exemplifies what trauma inflicts on memory: perforating it, it renders the testimonial narrative itself into a text that oscillates between the mechanic adherence to the details of horror and the collapse into the black holes of no-memory.

Notes

1 Quotes from *W, or the Memory of Childhood*, trans. David Bellos are reprinted by permission of David R. Godine, Publisher, Inc. Copyright © Georges Perec, 1987.
2 In this context, see the discussion of the letter x as the basis of a geometrical fantasy, in which the basic figure is the double V, whose many configurations form the major symbols of his childhood story (p. 77).
3 Here too, as in many other places in the book, there is a gap between the concrete and fictional facts: on the back of the photograph is written "1939", but when he describes the photograph he says: "I think it dates from 1938" (p. 49)
4 While recounting these memories in writing – he recalls an additional memory, and yet he does not change the number of memories to "four". Does he wish to maintain the sequence of the recollection as is? Or is this rather a conscious or unconscious attempt to undermine every fact and every attempt to constitute a linear sequence?

References

Amir, D. (2012). The inner witness. *International Journal of Psycho-Analysis*, 93, 879–896.

Amir, D. (2016). *On the lyricism of the mind: Psychoanalysis and literature*. London: Routledge.

Amir, D. (2017). Traumatic miss and the work of mourning. *fort da*, 23(2), 7–16.

Matte Blanco, I. (1975). *The unconscious as infinite sets. An essay in bi-logic*. London: Gerald Duckworth & Company Limited.

Perec, G. ([1975] 2010). *W or the memory of childhood*. (trans: D. Bellos). Boston, MA: D. R. Godine.

Chapter 3

The post-traumatic dyad

Agota Kristóf's *The Notebook*

Agota Kristóf's novel *The Notebook* (1997) follows the experiences of a pair of twins who, during an unspecified war, are left in the care of their grandmother whom they haven't met until then. Neither the geographical nor the historical location of the events is clear. It seems we are in Europe, sometime midways the twentieth century. The twins' grandmother is violent, ignorant, shrewd and cruel. The two children, at least as the story begins, are portrayed as her inverse: well educated, spoilt, intelligent. As the narrative proceeds, these extremes become surprisingly and disturbingly interwoven and entangled.

The Notebook consists of the twins' jointly written diary. Underlying its composition is a basic rule: the law of objectivity. This means that the text must describe facts rather than feelings and represent concrete details, not their subjective interpretations. The result is a dry account, lacking in emotional substance and devoid of a narrator's viewpoint. The use of the first person plural blurs the distance not only between self and other, but also between self and the horror out there. Thus, the twins turn evil into a form of survival: from being the helpless victims of the horror they become part of it.

Though the whole of the book is written in a metonymic mode its effect is psychotic. It reproduces a sense of alienation both from oneself and from the other, and metonymically enacts the sense of rupture in the causal chain of events and the sharp turn in the order of things; yet, at the same time, it creates a text that allows neither closeness nor distance. This is not a living testimony, but rather an account that attacks the very ability to bear witness. The narrators, who lose their unique voices to a mechanical anonymity of twinhood, are not two, or two-who-are-one: they are not even one.

The current chapter is dedicated to the special syntax of post-traumatic dyads (Amir, 2013) and the attack they perform on the "function of the witness" (Amir, 2012, 2014); to the way in which the "I" turns into "we" under the traumatic terror and to the de-subjectivization this "we" allows not only as an unavoidable side-effect but also as a mechanism of survival.

The book's opening sentence already announces what is to follow: "We arrive from the big town" (Kristóf, 1997, p.3). First of all, "we": neither "I", nor "I, who am called … and he, whose name is so and so …" – but "we": a tight, impregnable and alienated first person plural.

"Mother's eyes are red" (p. 3). According to the rule the twins imposed on themselves they must deal with the external facts rather than with what those facts arouse in them: with the surface of things, not with their inner world and its effect on their observations. This is the reason why they are not writing "Our mother is sad", or "Our mother is tired", but rather refer to the external fact of her red eyes. Their relation to the outside does not emerge from within but is rather directed from surface to surface. They do not interpret. They describe. Their first-person plural does not only constitute a buffer between each of them and every other person, but also between each of them and himself.

The dialogue between the mother and the grandmother suggests that the trauma at hand is already predisposed by an earlier, archaic trauma – that of the alleged murder of the children's grandfather by their grandmother, years ago. Thus, to save the twins' lives, the mother takes them back to the primary site of breakdown, to the place of her own deepest wound. The fact that the act of persecution and the act of rescue might take place in the same spot and featured by the same protagonist creates a kind of "schizophrenogenic double-bind" quite at the beginning of the plot.

Soon enough the twins acquire the rules of the new reality, manifesting themselves as expert survivors: they saw through the ladder to the attic, so their grandmother won't be able to climb it; they drill holes in the floor so as to be able to spy on the rooms of their grandmother and the officer who is a lodger in her house; they make a master key that fits all the locks in the house.

In their attic, they hide the notebook and a dictionary their father gave them, which they keep from the eyes of strangers. The notebook and dictionary may be seen as representing their attempt to translate to themselves the language of their new reality. But though they are able to sketch highly accomplished maps, their language, which stays alienated and descriptive, is very poor at making connections: instead of enabling thought it constitutes a kind of "attack on linking" (Bion, 1959), reducing speech to a mechanical act which bears no message of transformation.

The narrators' objective position never evolves into a reflective one:

> Grandmother is mother's mother. Before coming to live in her house, we didn't even know that mother still has a mother.
> We call her Grandmother.
> People call her the Witch. She calls us "sons of a bitch".
>
> (p. 8)

The twins neither mention any feelings nor ask any questions (Why, for instance, didn't they know about the existence of this grandmother? Why does she address them in that way?). They are not making any attempt to create a rich biographical continuity between their present life and their previous one. Instead, they mechanically assemble facts and details, their discourse gradually becoming a way of deploying thinking for survival.

At first, they refuse to help their grandmother with the chores. On the sixth day, they surrender:

> At the meal, Grandmother says:
> "Now you understand. You have to earn food and shelter."
> We say:
> "It's not that. The work is hard, but to watch someone working and not do anything is even harder, especially if it's someone old."
> Grandmother sniggers:
> "Sons of a bitch! You mean you felt sorry for me?"
> "No, Grandmother. We just felt ashamed."
>
> (p. 11)

At this point the twins still dwell within the moral world order. They give in to their grandmother, not in the name of the rules she has set, but in the name of the rules according to which they were raised. They give in to her, that is, by dint of the moral values which belong in their former world. Their grandmother, by contrast, speaks from the new world in which feelings and values are nothing but an obstacle. The difference between "feeling sorry for" and "feeling ashamed" is that "feeling ashamed" still maintains a self-reflective position. In this early interaction, thus, one can observe the confrontation between the twins' self-reflective position and their grandmother's flat and alienated one.

In an attempt to bear the physical pain, the twins evolve a survival method of their own: they hit and hurt each other in order to grow stronger. Each time they hurt themselves they say: "It doesn't hurt":

> After a while, we really don't feel anything anymore. It's someone else who gets hurt, someone else who gets burned, who gets cut, who feels pain.
>
> (p. 17)

This brings to mind Ferenczi's statement (1921) regarding the child who exiles him-or-herself from his or her own body to the point of experiencing the catastrophic event as something that happened to someone else. It also resonates with Laub's (2005) argument to the effect that we can only know our story as we tell it to an-other, or to an-other within us. Not only that the twins do not serve as "others" – their notebook, which they use to document what befalls them, does not constitute a symbolic other as well: they do not use it to tell their own story, but rather tell a story from which they are missing, one in which they are progressively present as objects rather than as subjects.

To inure themselves against the constant verbal abuse, they train themselves – much like their work on coping with physical pain – in verbally hurting each other until words can no longer inflict pain:

> But there are also the old words.
> Mother used to say to us:
> "My darlings! My loves! My joy! My adorable little babies!"
> When we remember these words, our eyes fill with tears.
> We must forget these words because nobody says such words to us now and because our memory of them is too heavy a burden to bear.
>
> (p. 21)

To overcome the hold that the old words have over them they create an exercise to subdue their influence:

> By force of repetition, these words gradually lose their meaning, and the pain they carry in them is assuaged.
>
> (ibid.)

What weakens the twins is not pain but tenderness. Where they encounter physical and mental pain they toughen up. But in the face of memory's tenderness, they find it hard to maintain their hermetic encapsulation. What dulls the impact of tenderness is repetition: the more they repeat the words that tie them to their past as well as to themselves, the weaker grows that link. They inure themselves not by avoiding what weakens them but by repeating it until it grows numb. In front of the catastrophic invasion, the only way to cope is by annihilating the experiencing subject along with the experience.

And indeed, the twins create "a post-traumatic autistic dyad" (Amir, 2013, 2014), one which erases both partners as subjects. Allowing the one to use the other by way of a partition that blocks out both the external and the internal world, this dyad generates one-dimensionality in place of three-dimensionality: a surface that is impenetrable to deep meaning. As the subjective existence of both its partners is expropriated, one may use the other, or parts of the other's presence, as something to fill holes with. So obliterated become the human qualities of the other, that this other may in fact come to serve as the thing that fills the hole of his or her own absence. And thus the other person can simultaneously be the absent person, the hole that opened up as a result of his or her absence, and the thing that blocks that hole, while this whole mechanical chain of events completely fails to be registered mentally (Amir, 2013, 2014).

The twins' description of a recollection from their first day at school, long before the war began, constitutes first evidence that this semi-autistic dyad was not just constituted by the present trauma but has primary roots:

Mother says: [...] they are one and the same person.

> Father raises his voice: Precisely, it isn't normal. They think together, they act together. They live in a different world. In a world of their own. [...] They're odd. You never know what they might be thinking.
>
> (pp. 22–23)

And indeed, when they are separated into different classrooms they faint:

> We are separated from one another by the whole length of the building. This distance between us seems monstrous, the pain is unbearable. It is as if they have taken half our bodies away. We can't keep our balance, we feel dizzy, we fall, we lose consciousness.
>
> (p. 23)

The importance of this episode lies in its foreshadowing the twins' mode of survival of the later trauma. Much like, at the start of their lives, they made up one unit in which neither of them existed separately, they eventually become one with the external catastrophe. This is not a simple case of identification with the aggressor, but rather a symbiosis with a malignant self-object (Kohut, 1971; Laub, 2005) which is the catastrophic object itself. Thus, they do not face the catastrophe as witnesses: they transform into it.

When they go to the stationery shop in order to buy paper and pencils, the shopkeeper yells at them that they speak "too correctly" (ibid.). Their elevated, accurate expression suits neither their age nor the external situation. They speak to but never speak with. The features of their language are, in that sense, autistic, generating a discourse that is syntactically exact but emotionally barren and rigid. Neither childish nor adult, their talk occurs outside of the rules of time and space, resembling the mechanical speech of a computer which while fed the exact rules, lacks the human interval that allows for error and thereby also for identification. In this context, the twins' insistence on learning, writing and calculating is especially intriguing. Rather than learning as a way to undergo change, they wrap and insulate themselves in survival-oriented knowledge serving as a "second skin" (Bick, 1968). Exactly as their language is the inverse of language, their learning is the inverse of learning: since they remove any subjective element from the process, they annihilate the possibility for the acquired material to be mentally metabolized:

> We have a very simple rule: the composition must be true. We must describe what is, what we see, what we hear, what we do.
>
> For example, it is forbidden to write, "Grandmother is like a witch"; but we are allowed to write "people call Grandmother the Witch".
>
> [...] We would write, "We eat a lot of walnuts," and not "We love walnuts," because the word "love" is not a reliable word [...]. Words that define feelings are very vague. It is better to avoid using them and stick to the description of objects, human beings, and oneself, that is to say, to the faithful description of facts.
>
> (p. 29)

Sticking to the objective is nothing but avoiding the subjective. Avoidance, that is, of anything that can generate specificity, depth or singularity, and thus cause pain. It is not just from the external and the internal world that the twins are protecting themselves. They also protect themselves from otherness by wholly undoing that otherness. We never know who of the two is writing the text. They have no names and, other than by way of a sort of exercise, they never address each other. The notebook does not register even one conversation between them. Their speech is not productive or fertilizing, it does not engender new thoughts and reflects no impregnation through language. It is rather a kind of rubbing of surfaces against one another. They cooperate perfectly, as though they were two bodies sharing one brain, one mind. But this turns them into a well-oiled emotionless machine. Thus, they are no more motivated by the wish to cause pain than they are motivated by the wish to avoid it. To each of these, it seems, they are equally indifferent. In a world in which humaneness is nothing but an obstacle, not only gestures of humaneness should be avoided but any other kind of human experience, too.

To this the chapter entitled "our neighbor and her daughter" presents a fascinating alternative. The neighbor's daughter (named Harelip) is not much older than the twins. Like them, she is coping with catastrophe: a miserable existence, a harelip, hunger, a mother who is, or pretends to be, both deaf and blind. She steals, she offers sexual services in exchange for money and attention, but unlike the twins, she preserves the wish to belong and to take part in human relations. When the twins offer her food, she shouts at them: "I don't want your fruit, your fish, or your milk! I can steal all that. What I want is for you to love me" (p. 32).

In one of the most shocking chapters of this novel, Harelip has sexual intercourse with the twins' dog. What is gripping about this scene is the gap it presents between her discourse and theirs: for though to her it is obvious that her acts testify to a disorder, which is why she checks whether they will still be her friends in spite of what they saw, nothing of the kind is obvious to the twins. Not only do they fail to be shocked, their description of the sexual scene is mechanical and alienated, with obvious reactions like disgust, arousal or even curiosity – completely missing. It seems that it is not only the written description that lacks an observing perspective, also the described experience itself goes without it. This is borne out by the fact that they have no difficulty whatsoever to continue being her friends after the event. So, if Harelip is located outside human society because the latter rejected her, they, on the contrary, no longer consider themselves part of it.

In the chapter "An Exercise in Deafness and Blindness", the twins undertake a series of mechanical exercises: while one of them covers his eyes with a handkerchief, the other blocks his ears with grass. Eventually, they no longer need any aids: "The one playing the blind man simply turns his gaze inward, and the deaf one shuts his ears to all sounds" (p. 40). This is an allegorical exercise that comes to symbolize their mode of survival. What they aim for is total control of everything: an autistic omnipotence within which they grow blind and deaf at will, lose touch with pain and with hunger and sever any link with their significant external objects as well as with their internal ones. Their ambivalence toward any show of tenderness is conspicuous wherever they encounter characters who approach them humanely: the servant, the postman, the cobbler. This ambivalence relates to the fact that these humane gestures do not only raise old memories but also trigger the twins' own humaneness and vulnerability. If the mother is their internal vulnerable object, then they must kill her in order to survive. In this sense, her concrete death, which occurs much later, repeats an internal scene that has already taken place.

In contrast with the one-dimensionality of the twins' witnessing position, the other figures in this text usually feature as duplicitous figures. This is the doubleness of care and exploitation. A good example is the priest's housekeeper who transforms the scene of the maternal washing of the twins into one of sexual abuse. Her sexual acts are performed on the children's bodies as she tells them how much she would have liked to be a mother to children just like them. This mention of the maternal function is not random. Do they regard their own mother, too, as an equivocal figure? Is this a hint suggesting that they feel that under the cover of protecting them their mother has actually abandoned them? Could it be that their later revenge on the housekeeper is not only related to her cruelty towards the hungry people who passed below her window, as the twins declare, but also to her representing the betrayal of their own mother?[1]

Like the housekeeper, the priest, too, takes an ambiguous parental role. He is portrayed on the one hand as a pedophile who has no qualms about exploiting Harelip to satisfy his sexual needs, but on the other hand, he talks with the twins about the Ten Commandments and wishes to pray for them. Again, like the housekeeper, the priest's character is not devoid of gentleness and nor is he categorically cruel. What the notebook seems to convey relates exactly to this traumatic contamination of kindness by cruelty, of care by abuse, of rescue by abandonment, which turns the entire environment into an uncanny one.

The twins' sado-masochistic relations with the military officer are described in a similar vein. In exchange for sexual services rendered, they are allowed to be in his room, to eat, to smoke and to listen to music. Later, when they are thrown into jail, they also gain his protection. Here, too, the relations are marked by the same duplicity that allows neither emotional link nor complete detachment. They understand the officer's sadomasochistic language as it fits naturally with their own mode of survival. It is no coincidence that they ignore the servant when he tries to warn them against the officer's exploitation. The twins hold on to their malignant objects and to malignancy itself as others hold on to love. The grandmother is the only one who does not betray them. Her sadism, stable and unchanging, is in that sense to be preferred over the mother's capricious tenderness. In the twins' eyes, it is easier to trust cruelty than to trust compassion since cruelty is much more stable and enduring.

When a government representative appears at the grandmother's house in order to compel the twins to return to school, they cheat the authorities by pretending that one of them is deaf and the other blind. The twins, here, might be seen to announce symbolically that the parental figures can no longer be restored. It is impossible to reinstate the order necessary for them to revert to being children. The law of the father has collapsed and along with it the capacity to constitute any functional hierarchy that allows care and responsibility. And indeed, in the course of the last chapters of this novel, the twins virtually annihilate the parental figures one by one, starting with their own mother (who dies as a result of a bombing when they keep her waiting at the entrance to the house), continuing with Harelip's mother, their grandmother and finally their father. Following the father's murder, the twins also separate from each other, when one of them crosses the border and the other stays on this side. Is their separation an attempt to generate a first-person singular – or is it an act of suicide? The end of the novel seems to allow each of these possibilities, and since in many ways the novel features psychic death as the one way to live – the double meaning of its end does not stray far.

The twins are in fact "doubles" (Freud, 1955 [1919]) rather than twins. This doubleness situates them in an uncanny environment in which they experience themselves quite from the beginning as half demons half humans, half children half adults, half mechanical half alive. In terms of the function of the inner witness (Amir, 2012, 2014) it seems that the post-traumatic dyad created by the twins was the result of an excess of primary violence (Aulagnier, 2001) along with the absence of a concrete or internalized third. From the start of their lives, they had to deal with two kinds of excessiveness: the excessiveness of the external, other twin, and the excessiveness of the unconscious murderous maternal legacy. These two kinds of excessiveness are nevertheless connected: the excessiveness of their twinhood positioned their mother in the role of the "third" instead of in the role of the "second" in the primary dyad. The problem was that the mother, stripped of the role of the "second", was unable to feature in the role of the "third" either. Because of her own traumatic legacy, she preferred to let them satisfy each other's needs, maybe as a way of saving them from her own unconscious wishes and phantasies. And since the father, for his part, kept his distance on account of their strangeness, hence remaining a stranger himself, the crucial developmental shift between the first person and the third person never occurred to undo the autistic dyadic perfection which the twins forged with each other, allowing no capacity for reflection or representation to emerge as a result.

The type of first person plural that they developed can bear witness to the outside but not to the inside, that is, to the external others but not to each other or to themselves. Hence the twins' uncanny ability to gauge another person's responses and to predict them on the basis of mere calculation, while lacking any ability to put themselves in the other's emotional position or to move between experiencing something and observing it. They are neither in the position of victims nor in the reflective position of witnesses. One might consider them "mechanical witnesses": witnesses who document events with almost digital precision, but neither leave their personal imprint on this documentation nor claim ownership of it. In this sense, they constantly reconstitute their experience as an "event without witness" (Felman, 1992): an event from which they, as witnesses, are absent.

Similarly to Camus' protagonist in *The Fall* (1956) and his refusal to bear witness to the woman's fall off the bridge – one may consider the twins' mode of witnessing a way of refusing for anything to enter them other than in the form of instrumental knowledge. Feelings, memories, yearnings – are constantly rejected. Detached knowledge is the only form that can enter or sustain the mind, floating in the inner mental space like a bizarre object: a thought without a thinker (Bion, 1962a, 1962b).

In that sense *The Notebook* presents us with one of the most subtle collapses of witnessing, carried out not by means of the fragmentation of the thinking apparatus itself but rather by means of the traumatic fissure between thought and thinker, between knowledge and the knowing I.

Note

1 Later we learn that their mother married another man during the war and gave birth to a baby girl.

References

Amir, D. (2012). The inner witness. *International Journal of Psycho-Analysis*, 93, 879–896.

Amir, D. (2013). The psychic organ point of autistic syntax. *Journal of Child Psychotherapy*, 39(1), 31–21

Amir, D. (2014). *Cleft tongue: The language of psychic structures*. London: Karnac Books.

Aulagnier, P. ([1975] 2001). (trans: A. Sheridan). *The violence of interpretation: From pictogram to statement*. East Sussex, UK: Bruner-Routledge.

Bick, E. (1968). The experience of the skin in early object relations. *International Journal of Psycho-Analysis*, 49, 484–486.

Bion, W. (1959). Attacks on linking. *International Journal of Psycho-Analysis*, 40, 308–315.

Bion, W. (1962a). *Learning from experience*. New York: Basic Books.

Bion, W. (1962b). The psycho-analytic study of thinking. *International Journal of Psycho-Analysis*, 43, 306–310.

Camus, A. ([1956] 2004). The fall (La Chute). In: A. Camus (Ed.), *The plague, The fall, exile and the kingdom, and selected essays*. (trans: J. O'Brien). New York: Everyman's Library.

Felman, S. (1992). Camus' the plague, or a monument to witnessing. In: S. Felman and D. Laub (Eds.), *Testimony: Crises of witnessing in literature, psychoanalysis, and history* (pp. 93—119). New York: Routledge.

Ferenczi, S. (1921). Psycho-analytical observations on tic. *International Journal of Psycho-Analysis*, 2, 1–30.

Freud, S. ([1919] 1955). The uncanny. In: J. Strachey (Ed.), *The standard edition of the complete psychological works of Sigmund Freud, volume XVII (1917–1919): An infantile neurosis and other works* (pp. 217–256). London: The Hogarth Press and the Institute of Psycho-Analysis.

Kohut, H. (1971). *The analysis of the self.* New York: International Universities Press.

Kristóf. A. (1997). *The notebook, the proof, the third lie*. (trans: A. Sheridan). New York: Grove Press.

Laub, D. (2005). Traumatic shutdown of narrative and symbolization. *Contemporary Psychoanalysis*, 41, 307–326.

Chapter 4

The center mode as opposed to the marginal mode

Yehiel Dinur (Ka-Tzetnik)'s *House of Dolls*

In his article "Body, Pleasure and Irony in the Representation of Suffering in the Holocaust" (2013), the historian Amos Goldberg discusses two literary ways in which pain experienced in the Holocaust has been expressed. He refers to the first as the "poetics of the bloc" and to the second as the "poetics of the slot". The poetics of the bloc is a poetics replete with pathos in which the text renders the unprocessed, unmitigated pain in its fullness and totality. The poetics of the slot, on the other hand, is characterized by an ironic mode and an attempt to crack the burden of suffering and undermine its all-embracing dominion. While the poetics of the bloc reenacts the excess of the Nazis' sadistic *jouissance*, the poetics of the slot escapes identification with the aggressor and uses irony and humor in order to cut a slot in the surplus fullness of the pain and regain in that way the power of subjectivity.

The current chapter uses Goldberg's distinction in order to put an edge on the difference between the testimonial narrative which undermines the subject qua witness, and whose poetics is the poetics of the bloc, based on generalizations and clichés – and the testimonial narrative which constitutes the subject qua witness, whose poetics cracks the fullness of pain in order to enable the crucial transition from matter to form, from experience to word.

The novel *House of Dolls* (1962) teems with excessive descriptions. These descriptions confer a double action upon the reader: while congesting the emotional space on the one hand, they also distance the reader from it on the other hand. Rina Dudai (2006) describes Ka-Tzetnik's characteristic use of poetic stratagems such as anaphora, hyperbole, tautology and dramatic punctuation, along with what she calls a "volcanic poetic language". These devices are deployed in order to create a textual congestion that arouses irrational emotions in the reader, thereby generating an effect of kitsch. Thus, for instance, Dudai demonstrates how repetitions create a "hypnotic effect" that causes an amplified sense of horror:

> The stillness exploded like a paper bag: **Shrieked** the barbed wires and **shrieked** the eyes strung out on them; **shrieked** the high heavens and **shrieked** the block rooftops.
>
> (Ka-Tzetnik, p. 205, emphasis added)

Dudai also demonstrates how the use of hyperboles makes the presented worldview total and absolute, with evil filling the world to the exclusion of all else:

> Harry stands amid **hordes** of bristling slaughter knives. **Everything** is red, crimson red. Around him, at him, **myriad** heads of drunken train guards guffaw through gaping maws. Knots of sparkling smoke belch and billow from the train chimneys towards the crimson-dark skies.
>
> (p. 18, emphasis added)

The novel's typical use of dramatic punctuation marks – like dashes, question marks at the end of rhetorical questions, exclamation marks and three dots (a means of rhetorical heightening which is particularly frequent in Ka-Tzetnik's novels in general) – serves the same purpose. All these devices testify to what Dudai refers to as "unrestrained heightened emotional activity", something further enhanced by the novel's tendency to use a metaphoric of volcanic activity, achieving in that way an amplifying, cosmic effect by describing the experience of the Holocaust in terms of natural disaster. These rhetorical methods bear out the "bloc poetics" described by Goldberg. They are employed in order to attain one purpose: the amplification of emotional congestion to such a degree that any aesthetic distance is destroyed, paralyzing the reader's judgment as well as his or her "position of the witness" (Amir, 2012, 2014).

Thus, for example, the second chapter opens with a saccharine poetic description, quoted from Daniela's (the female protagonist of *House of Dolls*) diary, of her vacation excursions across the city. This is immediately followed by a dark, somber description, replete with horror, of a nightmare she had the night before the fateful excursion from which she never returned home. Both the nature descriptions and the details of her dream are saturated with pathos, and moreover hyperbolic and extreme in their powerfully contrasting relation to one another:

> The moon shaft no longer lay on the table. It now gleamed sharp and angular through a corner of the open window directly at her head, appearing like a long, steel-sharp javelin piercing her temples, and pinned in the wall beside her bed.
>
> (p .18)

The same hyperbolic poetics is manifest in the description of Daniela's parting from her father and brother. Here, too, a great effort is made to inflate the drama of parting through the description of her father running after her to the train station in order to give her the locket she has forgotten at home, taking along with him her younger brother who refuses to part from her. Immediately following is a description of the train carrying a machine gun whose long barrel is aimed towards the sky. All this anticipates the impending catastrophe which will cut right through Daniela's peaceful life.

Alongside the content-related anticipation, the text also renders the poetics I would like to outline here in terms of its form: by presenting the good as radical perfection, evil is taken to its ultimate extreme. This poetics comes to induce a reader response marked by an almost absolute splitting between the innocence and the goodness of before and the ensuing evil and loss of trust thereafter. In that way it obviates the reader's autonomous capacity to anticipate what is about to take place; so explicit and telling are the omens, and conveyed by a narrator so omniscient, that they neutralize the reader's own position of the witness. It is as if the poetics of the block rams the information down the reader's throat, thus doing the work on their behalf while depriving them of both the need and freedom to take a stance of their own.

One of the greatest dangers lurking in the territory of excess is the danger of collusion. Shmuel Erlich (2013) writes that an allegedly shared trauma might at times push the patient and therapist in the therapeutic process towards a deceptive sense of solidarity which undermines the very therapeutic work. One may say that as in the case of therapeutic work with trauma, where a warning light should go on as soon as there is mutual satisfaction between patient and therapist – when mutual satisfaction occurs between writer and reader regarding the catastrophic aspects of the text one should be forewarned against the danger of indulgent collusion with the aggressor created by this text. Indulgence in the traumatic experience undermines the possibility of bearing witness to it. Ka-Tzetnik's saturated pathos therefore activates in relation to the reader the very thing to which it testifies: the attack on the subject's autonomy and his or her freedom to reclaim their witnessing position as their own.

Whereas the "slot" poetics activates thinking and in that way brings the witness to life, the "bloc" poetics, through its unbearable congestive quality, leads to detachment. What distances the reader in the bloc poetics may well be his or her own *jouissance* which arouses unconscious resistance to the text, as might be the case in the following quotation:

> Here it is, life! Here! Poised on the threshold of his body, like a bird at the portal of its ravaged nest before taking wing. Who is so blind that could not now tangibly see the sheer, naked life of man? It now pauses outside him, as if wanting to cast one last glance at the place it is about to leave, forever. [...] To the sick bay had he come. Two hours he stood in line. It had given him no rest. Please, would the Physician help make it possible for him to cry. [...] But where, in the German camp, at the last moment, are you to get a tear? [...] In his last moment – a tear! Who could now get him a tear?
>
> (pp. 98–99)

The pathos that characterizes this quotation prompts a reader response that resembles the phenomenon of reaction-formation: the text is so emotionally demanding that the reader collapses in so far as he or she is an empathetic listener, becoming a distant, critical recipient who is forced to impose the slots that are absent from the testimonial text itself.

> In the sick bay everything is spick and span. Harry[1] is depressed and heavy hearted. On the table, the empty bottles are arrayed in straight rows along the wall. The upstretched necks of the bottles claw at his brain. They bristle like bayonet points, spring out of the neat rows, up and down, up and down, and stab under his scalp. [...] Stillness. Idyll. An idyll to drive a man out of his mind.
>
> (p. 101)

The parallel between the sterility of the camp's hospital room and the sterile mechanism underlying the Nazi regime's methods of extermination is achieved here by means of extremely simplistic figurative methods; the resulting text requires no "work" on the part of the reader: indeed there seems to be an implied demand that such work will not take place. The excessive testimonial mode demonstrated here dissolves the reader as a subject: not by starving him or her by means of detachment (as Kristóf does, for example), but by gagging him or her with ready-made food.

Daniela's shocking encounter with her neighbor to the board is "served up" to the reader in the same manner:

> Her neighbor clutches the crust with two fleshless hands. With flaming eyes she examines the crust from all sides. The rusty tea can stands between her thighs. She throws open a mouth full of enormous poised teeth. It looks as if the teeth would swallow the crust down in one bolt. But the teeth just embrace the bread, touch it and let it out whole. [...] The teeth bite into the bread again and again, embrace it with ecstatic fervor, and once more release it – whole. Yet the black crust in the hands grows smaller, smaller, until nothing is left of it. But the teeth don't let up baring themselves and biting voraciously into the grimy, fleshless palms where earlier there had been a piece of bread. When she is tired of lapping at the memory of the bread, her eyes shifted towards the portion still lying untouched in Daniela's hands. The eyes sank into the black patch of bread and sucked and swallowed it from afar.
>
> (pp. 142–143)

Here the reader is made to participate passively in a ritual of horror, without being afforded the possibility to regulate the aesthetic distance from what is taking place and to determine his or her own response. In contrast to the dynamics marking the encounter with the writings of Perec – the reader of Ka-Tzetnik's book resists their own annihilation by distancing and alienating themselves.

Surprisingly or not, what fascinates in Ka-Tzetnik's text relates to events taking place far from the hyperbolic arena of overt rhetoric. Among the various characters surrounding Daniela, two are especially fascinating: the first is a possibly autistic, or maybe post-traumatic girl from

Oswiecim[2]. This ageless girl uncannily anticipates approaching Aktionen[3] and vanishes each time until the danger has passed. The other character is Fella, who generously shares the bread she obtains in return for the sexual services she provides. These two characters serve as each other's mirror image: while the possibly autistic girl saves her body but sacrifices her mind, Fella is willing to sacrifice her body for the purpose of saving her psyche.

Thus, while Ka-Tzetnik portrays Daniela and Harry, his declared protagonists, as tragic heroes who are led passively and helplessly to their inevitable end, the secondary narrative of Fella presents the possibility not only of actual survival but also of an alternative testimonial mode to the excessive writing he dedicates to his two heroes. Fella, who observes the traumatic realm from a distance that allows her to describe the events without collapsing into the rhetoric of excessive description – exemplifies the use of the metaphoric mode of testimony, which enables her though being part of the traumatic scene to also depart from it. While situating his two heroes in a text which is both addicted to itself and enslaved to its own set of images – Ka-Tzetnik renders the supporting characters (the girl from Oswiecim and Fella) a different voice. While the leading characters collapse under the burden of bloc poetics, the marginal characters extricate themselves from the excessive mode and manage to smuggle moments of metaphoric testimony through the cracks in this compressed text.

Thus for example in the following text:

> When Fella got to the Joy Division, she immediately saw there was bad business ahead for her. She, Fella, of the Jewish town of Radno, isn't going to be able to live in the same four walls with Elsa of Dusseldorf. One of them's got to give up: either – she, or – Elsa. The place just isn't big enough for both of them. [...] For never so much as now did Fella crave so to live for the day of liberation – of revenge. That being the case, she first has to get out from under Elsa's thumb. [...] Fella isn't letting Elsa squash her like a worm. She just won't be able to hold herself back. She'll fly off the handle and paste into the "Frankenstein" of Dusseldorf and really bitch things up – not only for herself but for all the Joy Division girls clear down through the last transport.
>
> (p. 194)

How different is this text, replete with humor and irony, from Daniela's pathos-saturated text relating to the same person:

> To the right of each girl marched a malefactress with a solemn, festive bearing, like a bridesmaid escorting a bride to the canopy. Elsa's slashed cheek looked from the distance as though half a mask had slipped from her face. The flesh between the crude stitchings now flushed blood red, appearing like a wound sawed into the flesh. The other half-face was taut, festive, solemn. The boot tops sparkled their Sabbath best on her feet, and near her right boot dangled the tail of her braided knout.
>
> (p. 204)

Thus, Ka-Tzetnik might be said to launch from the overt text a covert one, carrying a hidden message. The message is that the task of survival, and the act of testifying even more so, can be deposited only within those who have access to the poetics of the slot, that is, those who are able to move between the different modes of testimony from a position of inner freedom.

As Harry continues to sink into an exhausting, self-righteous chatter, his poetics eliminate his own stance as a credible witness. Indeed Ka-Tzetnik's hero reaches the moment of salvation (the moment of his meeting with Daniela) reduced to *Muselmann* condition, producing an indiscriminate jumble of hallucinations, fragments of memory and fragments of thought (p. 238). The attempt to create a musical "stretto", that is, to compress the traumatic plot till it overflows, brings *jouissance* to its perverse peak. Here as well, the parallel between the content-related conscious and the form-related unconscious is interesting: while the content-related aspects of the text deal with the collapse of the witness, that is, with Harry losing his mind, the form-related aspects make the reader, too, lose his or her mind in the sense that their perverse congestion attacks his or her very ability to process them.

Dudai (2015) quotes Kulka's (1996) discussion of the conditions for a poetics of kitsch:

> [...] kitsch does not risk taking an avant-garde stance, or adopting a style that is not universally acceptable. It comes into being only after innovation has become canonical and fossilized. [...] Kitsch always

> appeals to the broadest common denominator, and it is always utterly clear: nothing is left to the imagination. [...] kitsch does not enrich our repository of associations in respect to the described themes and objects, nor does it exploit the artistic possibilities of innovatively developing the structure or modes of expression. Kitsch hews close to stereotype. The subject must be presented in a standard and schematic fashion, with no individuality. Kitsch does not enhance our sensitivity, nor does it help us to make more refined distinction and discriminations. Kitsch often obstructs real emotions [...] it provides a simulacrum of the emotion that erodes and degrades the capacity to feel that emotion.
>
> (Kulka in Dudai, 2015, p. 21)

This goes hand-in-hand with the central claim of this chapter: rather than enabling thinking the excessive mode of testimony negates it, using the most deceptive means, attracting and seducing the reader into the swamp of non-thinking.[4] Ka-Tzetnik's language is a saturated language, one that does not enable transformation but rather undermines both testimony and witness. This is not the rich poetics of mourning, but rather one that creates an addictive fetish-like ritual, separating the witness both from the traumatic experience as well as from his own subjectivity.

Rina Dudai distinguishes, following Freud and LaCapra, between the poetics of acting-out and the poetics of working-through: acting-out is a subject's impulsive action that establishes the traumatic past within the present, reviving it without the ability to observe the conflicts it involves. The subject of acting-out recalls nothing of what has been repressed and forgotten, and therefore acts in light of the implicit memory without being aware of the origin of the act and its meaning. In the poetics of working-through, on the other hand, the subject forms an emotional insight that enables a type of aesthetic distance from which it is possible to understand, to see, to express in words and control what was previously not seen, not understood, neither defined nor conceived. Restraint becomes an expression of homeostatic balances that enable the traumatic experience to be preserved as a text, and in this sense serves as a measure of the text's metaphoric capacity to control the destructive forces, contain them and engender a new order on their basis.

However, for Dudai it is exactly the kitsch substances, with their poetics of acting-out, that preserve traces of the unconscious. Kitsch fulfills the aesthetic lie in order to nevertheless express, or cry out, the horror of the negative sublime.

Contrary to Dudai, I believe that the poetics of kitsch does not allow for the traumatic Real to be exposed but rather blocks any access to it. The rhetoric of excess freezes the very thing to which it wishes to bear witness. Ka-Tzetnik's testimony is in this sense based on the unconscious attempt to annihilate the witness. It comes as no surprise, therefore, that the book concludes with the collapse of both witnesses: Harry is taken back to the sick-bay where until recently he served as the camp medic and where he now lies terminally ill, while Daniela takes her own life after depositing her diary with Fella. The fact that neither Harry nor Daniela reaches the end of this journey in order to bear witness to their own experiences is related to the manner in which Ka-Tzetnik's poetics unconsciously undermines itself, causing its witnesses to collapse and negate their own testimony.

This is why Daniela's diary can only be deposited with Fella, whose poetics is a metaphoric one, marked by irony and reflective distance. Fella, the prostitute who from the start was not meant to evoke any identification, is precisely for this reason spared identificatory excess. This is why she survives as a witness: the aesthetic and emotional distance maintained in the author's relation to her saves, paradoxically, her very capacity to testify, both to herself and to the others.

Notes

1 Daniela's older brother.
2 The original Polish name of Auschwitz.
3 Mass deportations.
4 Hanna Arendt (1963) in her *Eichmann in Jerusalem: A Report on the Banality of Evil*, discussed Eichmann's consistent use of "stock phrases and self-invented clichés" as well as his reliance on "officialese" (Amtssprache) and the euphemistic Sprachregelung which made the implementation of Hitler's policies "somehow palatable". This might point to the similarity already hinted earlier between the language of the perpetrator and the language of the victim who unconsciously identifies with him.

References

Amir, D. (2012). The inner witness. *International Journal of Psycho-Analysis*, 93, 879–896.

Amir, D. (2014). *Cleft tongue: The language of psychic structures*. London: Karnac Books.

Arendt, H. (1963). *A report on the banality of evil*. New York: The Viking Press.

Dudai, R. (2006). Kitsch ve trauma – Mikre mivchan: beit ha-boobot me-et K. Tsetnick. [Kitsch and trauma – Test case: House of Dolls by Ka-tsetnick.]. *Mikan*, 6, 125–142.

Dudai, R. (2015). Pain and pleasure in poetic representations of the past. In: A. Goldberg and H. Hazan (Eds.), *Marking evil: Holocaust memory in the global age* (pp. 233–265). New York: Berghahn Books.

Erlich, H. S. (2013). *The couch in the marketplace: Psychoanalysis and social reality*. London: Karnac.

Goldberg, A. (2013). Body, pleasure and irony in the representation of suffering in the Holocaust. In: O. Meital and S. Stav (Eds.), *Pain in the flesh*. Beer-Sheva, Israel: Ben-Gurion University of Negev Press.

Ka-Tzetnik. (1962). *House of dolls*. (trans. M. M. Khan). Great Britain: Panther.

Kulka, T. (1996). *Kitsch and Art*. Philadelphia, PA: Pennsylvania State University Press.

Chapter 5

The traumatic lacuna as the negative possession of the other

Aharon Appelfeld's "Bertha"[1]

"Bertha" by Aharon Appelfeld (1994) is one of the few literary works in which the Muselmann-psychotic mode is both described and enacted. This is the story of Max, a man in his prime, who lives with an ageless woman who suffers from an undefined syndrome that seems, but is not overtly declared, to be a blend of retardation and autism. She was handed to him during the war: a child nobody could bear and whom he could not leave behind. The short story follows Max's attempt to part from Bertha and to establish an intimate relationship and a life of his own, an attempt that comes to a vague ending when she is transferred to some medical or psychiatric institution where she possibly dies.

The story opens with an exposition of the characters and their types of movement or non-movement:

> In winter, he would return. Perspiring, a knapsack on his back, he would bring with him the fresh scent of worlds unknown here. His comings and goings were quiet. You never knew whether he was happy to leave or happy to return. Inside, in the small room, life remained unchanged. Bertha would sit on the floor, knitting. It seemed as if the passing of years did not touch her. She remained just as he had left her in summer, small, dwarfish even, and quite unaltered.
>
> (p. 149)

While Max is characterized by an ostensibly linear movement, outwards and back – Bertha's movement is circular, preserving both herself and her surroundings in a state of stagnation. The meeting of the two constitutes a repetitive ritual:

> Bertha would light the stove, and Max, like a weary traveler, would sink into a long slumber that lasted through the winter. Only in early spring would he stretch himself, saying, "Well, Bertha, it's time I was on my way".
>
> (p. 149)

Ostensibly, Bertha marks the still, unchanging point in Max's changing world. As the story develops, however, it becomes clear that Max's seemingly linear movement is no more than a variation on Bertha's circular movement. Like her, he moves in routine tracks and fixed seasons, back and forth along an unchanging route, circling around her still point:

> Between naps he would try, half maliciously, half affectionately, to discuss his plans for her. The conversations were full of tears and laughter, and in the end everything remained as before. Max would leave on his travels, and Bertha remained behind. And so the seasons changed, one year followed another, a sprinkling of white appeared at Max's temples, [...] but Bertha remained as she was, small and dwarfish, these qualities becoming more pronounced, perfected as it were.
>
> (p. 149)

Every aspect of their lives related to movement, development and accumulation is gradually revealed as illusory. On the surface there is a movement to and from the house; a conversation pertaining to Max's plans for Bertha occurs, discussions are held, feelings are expressed, but in effect, these actions are performed solely in the service of repetition.

> At first, he had tried, firmly enough, to put her into an institution for girls. He had even had a few preliminary meetings with the headmistress of the institution, who had turned out to be a strong woman with piercing eyes whom he couldn't stand from the very first meeting. The plan, of course, came to nothing. [...] There had been one other serious attempt to find her what might be called a suitable living arrangement. [...] Bertha returned the next day, her eyes full of tears, and the matter was closed. Soon afterward he began to travel. Max left, hoping

> that within a year people would make some arrangements for her, or that she herself would find some way out, when after a year, upon returning to his room, he found her sitting on the floor among skeins of wool, half knitting, half playing [...].
>
> (p. 150)

Max's and Bertha's identities are interwoven. While he is in charge of the vivid and developing part – she holds the eternal, frozen time of the traumatic wound on his behalf. Bertha is Max's traumatic lacuna. This lacuna is the load that Max can neither leave behind nor move forward with. Fleeing from and returning to it, this is both his source of guilt and no less what stands between him and the very possibility of a new life.

Bertha and Max are suspended between life and death, between an arrested childhood and a never-achieved maturity. He leaves and returns in the same manner that she knits and un-knits; in effect, she outwardly manifests what he bears within. It is not by chance that he cannot stand the piercing eyes of the institution's headmistress: it seems that her eyes penetrate their hermetic dyad, perhaps even expose their secret alliance. Although on the face of it Bertha is the one who has not been able to accept any external solution – Max, too, cannot let go of Bertha and what she stands for.

> Several years passed – five years, or more. The passage of time became blurred, especially since there were no innovations. Life went on its lazy routine, devouring time. [...] Between naps he would sit and watch her, as if he were observing his own life.
>
> (p. 150)

Bertha serves as an external reflection of Max's inner world ("Closed, encased in a hard shell, she dragged after him like a dead weight, and sometimes like a mirror wherein his life was reflected" – p. 150). Like her, he exists between naps, in a state of semi-consciousness, allowing time to blur and life to consume its potential for renewal.

> Sometimes, he went haunted by the old question of his purpose in life. What was he to do with her, or what was she going to do? It was her duty to think of it – she must not be a perpetual burden on him.
>
> (p. 150)

The wording 'haunted by the old question of his purpose in life' is especially interesting in this context: the question of action and purpose is attributed to what Appelfeld calls "the old world", the world prior to the traumatic fracture. In the terminology of the old world, the question of purpose is meaningful, entailing crucial practical conclusions. After the fracture, however, the old world's dispensation is no longer valid. This is why the moments when Max is overcome by the "question of purpose", are experienced as haunting moments that he should renounce. In a world whose order has collapsed there is no point in asking questions about purpose, and taking action aimed towards a purpose is nothing but a form of self-deception.

Bertha, who is situated outside the linear continuum of place and time, is the only one who deceives neither herself nor others:

> She was stubbornly loyal, another quality that was not quite human. All summer long she would sit and knit fantastic patterns in strange colors. [...] They were not sweaters. A dumb smile would appear on her face at the sight of the patterns. In the end she would unravel them and then the same wool would appear again on the needles, year after year. The tape measure he brought her was no help, since she did not seem to understand what it was for.
>
> (pp. 150–151)

Bertha is the very signifier of trauma: too massive to be represented through language, too diffuse to be situated within the coordinates of common perception (space, time, causality). Max's rigid timetable alone provides her with an outline, a frame circumscribing her vague existence. And she, in turn, serves as a permanent object, a kind of beacon or point of reference in relation to which he can move back and forth. In this sense, her knitting serves a double purpose: it binds him to her with the twines of her wool ("I'm knitting for Maxie" – pp. 150–151), but it also creates a chronic, compulsive ritual of weaving and unraveling of the psychic envelope.

This chronic weaving and unraveling is in itself a form of testimony. Greek mythology offers quite a few stories related to the craft of weaving and unraveling: Athena the weaver, the goddesses responsible for the thread of life and death, and Penelope, weaving and unweaving, for the length of Ulysses' absence. One of the less known of these weaving characters is Philomela who was brutally raped by the king of Thrace. He cut out her tongue and imprisoned her in order to prevent her from testifying to his deeds. Distraught, she wove the horrific story into a tapestry which she sent to her sister, who deciphered the story and released her from her bondage. For Bertha, as for Philomela, the act of knitting is an act of bearing witness. However, while Philomela transmits a "full testimony" – even if it is through images rather than words – in Bertha's case, testimony does not concern the traumatic event itself, but rather the traumatic lacuna created as a result of it, a lacuna that by its very essence cannot be woven into a narrative. In this sense, the unknitting, no less than the knitting, tells her story.

For both Max and Bertha, the traumatic lacuna has become a type of negative possession (Amir, 2012, 2014), which serves as an existential anchor while at the same time consuming the entire existential space.

> From the day that they had reached this country, oblivion had overcome her. Her memory froze at a certain point. You couldn't make her disclose anything from the past, nor was she capable of absorbing anything new. "Some pipe is stopped up." This feeling, oversimplified as it might be, remained a sort of certainty that he could not doubt, feeling as he did that something was clogged up in him, too.
>
> (p. 151)

Max and Bertha both exist in the shadow of a memory they cannot recall. It is the necessity not to remember, together with the inability to forget (for it is not possible to forget what one cannot remember) that keeps them together. Bertha has become sealed in a way that allows nothing to come out (in the form of a narrative or memory) or to enter (in the form of development and change). One could say she has retreated into an autistic state – into a position that uses the other as a psychic (as well as somatic) skin and forms a relationship with him solely through the friction of external surfaces. Max – like her – loses his sense of time and reality in her presence. Communication between them therefore resides in a frozen present rather than containing past and future; it is not an occurrence which takes place between two separate subjects but rather a repetitive echoing of each other's words, devoid of any impregnation or development.

Donald Meltzer (1975) uses the term "adhesive identification" for a sort of defensive adhesiveness of one person to another, a gesture related, rather than to love, to the attempt to lessen the subject's anxiety of disintegration.

Thus, the subject adopts the facial expressions of the other, his or her body movements as well as vocal attributes – all in order to use this external surface and the visual, musical and tactile characteristics of this surface – as if they were his or her own. Mimicry of this type consists of the "adhesion" of scraps from the surface of the other to the subject's own frail surface, in an attempt to use the other's "patches" of identity in order to stitch together one's own perforated identity. This is not an internalization of the other (in fact there is no sense of an interior into which something can be "taken in"); rather the contrary: since the psychic envelope is felt as perforated and the experience is one of leaking out of it – one creates an incessant friction with the other, which has the double purpose of preserving both the other and the self as incessantly present. This can also take place through the repetitive friction with the language of the other, in a way that does not constitute a real conversation but creates a mechanic and circular discourse, as in the case of Max and Bertha:

> "Isn't it beautiful today ..." he tried.
> "Beautiful," she said.
> "Isn't it beautiful today ..." he tried again.
> "Beautiful," she said.
>
> (p. 152)

The conversation serves as a type of negative possession: instead of letting new thoughts in, it turns speech into a repetitive, compulsive ritual, based on the profound refusal of any type of change, which is experienced as catastrophic (Bion, 1967). This repetition should not be understood in terms of its content, but rather as a mechanical, magical act of union centering on the very *need to say* rather than on any specific content. This is a sort of crude pleading, a voice that confirms simultaneously, through repetition, the existence of the plea's addressee and addresser, like a ball that, when thrown at a wall and bounces back, confirms the existence of both the thrower and the wall.

The torturous catch of adhesive identification is exactly this: it posits the other as so close, so identical, that he or she is no longer experienced as an-other, and therefore cannot provide the consolation that an-other's presence may provide. The only way to extricate oneself from this snare is through the act of mourning. Within the trauma's continuous present, however, neither the act of mourning nor the act of representation are possible.

> Then came the time that seemed ordained to bring this feeling to a head; a decision had to be taken. His fellow workers saw the need to interfere. Max needed a wife. It started, as these things usually do, as a joke. Later they fixed up a date for him – with a typist at the plant. [...] They didn't speak about Bertha. But with her feminine intuition she discovered it in a roundabout way. He could have said that she was retarded, that she would soon be put in an institution. [...] But he couldn't put it that way; something stopped him from saying the words. Sometimes your cunning betrays you, and you are suddenly left naked and ashamed. At those moments you are as vulnerable as a bare neck at the change of the seasons.
>
> (p. 153)

Mitzi's (the typist) alien, external gaze entering Max and Bertha's dyad constitutes a catastrophic penetration. Not only because of her concrete demand that he separate from Bertha, but also, or mostly, because of the deeper significance of this demand, namely that Max leave behind the part that Bertha both represents and holds for him.

> But the secret weighed on him. Was it still a secret? He had told everything. He thought he had exhausted the matter. That is how it seemed to him [...]. Late at night, during the second shift when the storehouse was empty, he suddenly felt that he was still carrying the secret within him. If only he could give it a name, he would feel easier; but the name eluded him.
>
> (p. 154)

The secret, so it seems, bears no relation to the real bond with Bertha ("Maybe she's yours; you can tell me, I won't blame you; things like that happened during the war" – p. 155), but rather to what constitutes the deep alliance between them in the first place: that "thing" that is not to be named, not because the name is shameful in itself – but because the name belongs in the symbolic order, while the "thing" dwells in the territory of the traumatic Real which refuses the very possibility of naming.

It is no coincidence that there is no institution to which Bertha could belong: neither a psychiatric institution nor any kind of other arrangement. The traumatic lacuna cannot be attributed in the terms of a common understanding, nor can it be included in any existing frame of reference. It is, in a sense, necessary to create a new language for it. Yet the need to create such a language, i.e. "to call Bertha by name", arises only when separation from her is forced upon Max. Or perhaps the opposite is correct: in order to be able to separate from her, he needs to be able to call her by name:

> His head was empty of all thoughts. He wasn't sure for what he had come. […] 'Bertha', he said. It was the biggest word that he could cut out of his heart; it seemed that only once had he called her that way, once at a Gentile woman's in Zivorka, after the big hunt when he was forced to leave her.
>
> (p. 156)

The capacity to call by name must derive from a position of estrangement. Yet Max cannot be estranged from Bertha, for rather than a separate entity she is the gaping abyss lurking within him:

> It was the same head, with the same tangled hair. A small, warm body that needed nothing, that was beyond patience, beyond any change that might come. […] you couldn't call it stupidity, idiocy, or any similar names called to mind by that strangeness. It was something different, something that a man like Max couldn't give a name to, but could feel.
>
> (p. 156)

Bertha is an element that is alien to the human ("She was a princess, a devil, a gypsy, something that could not be contained in any human measure" – p. 156), just as the traumatic lacuna is alien to common perceptual categories such as continuity and causality. She is not "estranged", but rather "the stranger" as such. In the conversation between Max and Bertha, in which he tries in vain to explain to her that they must part, she utters his name again and again:

> "Max!" she said. Not a muscle moved in her face.
> "I came early this time." He too was unable to utter another word.
> […]
> "Max!" said Bertha, as if cutting short his confession.
>
> (p. 156)

In effect, everything that happens from this point onwards is enfolded in the act of their calling each other by name: the element whose name is "Bertha" is about to be separated from the element whose name is "Max". This parting, which fails to take into account the primordial entwinement and interdependence of their identities, threatens to turn – through their calling by name – from a scene of creation into a scene of reversal back to the primordial chaos.

Bertha develops a burning fever and is rushed to hospital:

> The casualty ward in the hospital was full, but they made room for her. [...] They told him that he must leave. The gate closed behind him. At that moment he could remember nothing. His eyes saw, his heart fumbled, the tips of his fingers were tingling. Inside the cavity of his skull, something floated as in a heavy fluid. [...] 'Can't I remember anything at all? My memory is gone.' [...] There was no connection between one thought and another. It was as if they had frozen in one of his arteries. His body was working properly and you could hear the gentle pulse within it. [...] Nothing came to him, not a single detail that would lead him on or connect anything. His eyes saw, and he could make out everything, still enlarged, as it had seemed to him before. But he couldn't remember a thing.
>
> (pp. 157–158)

The moment Max separates from Bertha, he himself becomes Bertha: an intact body whose stream of consciousness has come to a halt, unable to connect between one detail and another so as to create a sequence of memory. At the moment of parting, the lacuna that thus far had borne the name "Bertha", or that had been deposited in Bertha, takes up residence in Max. In a process akin to a sort of inverted birth, Max parts from "Bertha" the object and for the first time internalizes Bertha as a representation of his own traumatic lacuna:

> Was it Bertha, or only a vision? [...] Again you went out to search for her the way you searched for her in the forest, the way you searched for yourself in the street. You just found details; you couldn't see her, just as you couldn't see yourself.
>
> (p. 159)

In doing so, however, the hitherto frozen memory thaws and becomes his own:

> Slowly, like a sharp stimulus, memory started ebbing back, around the thin tubes of his temples. He clutched his head afraid that it would burst. [...] Now he was already in the realm of the forms. Reality, as it were, shed its skin; all he felt was a kind of familiarity, as if he were being drawn – he did not know toward what; to the blue color, to the trees or to the stray dog that chanced to be there. He did not see Bertha. She had become something that could no longer be called Bertha.
>
> (p. 158)

The description of his being drawn to the colors of nature resembles a moment in which colors and sounds slowly seep back into a film that so far screened as a silent, black and white movie. Max's awakening from his state of drowsy consciousness and his return to life is related to the transformation of Bertha from "someone" to "something": "Something that could no longer be called Bertha", but may hold the chance to finally assume its real name.

Having regained an inner world and mental life, Max is flooded by dreams:

> The dream became full of ceremonies. Sometimes she was handed over to him and sometimes a delegation came to claim her from him [...]
>
> (p. 159)

It is not by chance that these dreams shift between experiencing Bertha as a burden he cannot remove and an asset he refuses to give up. The traumatic lacuna's power is twofold: it empties – but in doing so it also produces the fullest witness. It is simultaneously experienced as an abyss as well as a possession, as something that both nullifies and organizes psychic existence.

Bertha is the representation of the *Muselmann* testimonial mode: unconnected to the trauma (in terms of memory), she cannot distance herself from it (in terms of reflective language). She stands between Max and the traumatic lacuna, defending him against its negative power, but at the same time preventing him from observing that lacuna and turning it from a negative possession into a possession. Her *Muselmann* mode enables Max to function within a metonymic mode of testimony, thus to create a continuous, albeit non-reflective existential sequence. But it stands between him and the metaphoric mode. The only way his existence can become three-dimensional is for Max to be the owner of his traumatic lacuna, which has so far been deposited in Bertha. Only by adopting this lacuna as an internal object he may restore the ability to remember together with the capacity to forget, or to maintain a language that survives the "bowels of hell", as Agamben writes (2002, p. 162), along with "a speaker who remains beyond it".

Note

1 "Bertha" by Aharon Appelfeld. Copyright © Aharon Appelfeld, 1962, used by permission of The Wylie Agency (UK) Limited. English translation Copyright © Institute for the Translation of Hebrew Literature. First published in Israel 1965. Published here by arrangement with The Institute for The Translation of Hebrew Literature.

References

Agamben, G. (2002). *Remnants of Auschwitz: The witness and the archive*. (trans: D. Heller-Roazen). New York: Zone Books.

Amir, D. (2012). The inner witness. *International Journal of Psycho-Analysis*, 93, 879–896.

Amir, D. (2014). *Cleft tongue: The language of psychic structures*. London: Karnac Books.

Appelfeld, A. (1994). "Bertha". (trans: T. Zandbak). In: M. Teichman and S. Leder (Eds.), *Truth and lamentation: Stories and poems on the Holocaust* (pp. 149–159). Urbana and Chicago, IL: University of Illinois Press.

Bion, W. R. (1967). Catastrophic change. Unpublished paper.

Meltzer, Donald. (1975). Adhesive identification. *Contemporary Psycho-Analysis*, 11, 289–310.

Chapter 6

Transcending the traumatic real

Six variations in six stories by Ida Fink

Ida Fink's writings present a number of different attempts to constitute a point of view that transcends the traumatic Real. This chapter is dedicated to eight of her short stories, illuminating in each one of them a different variation of the theme of psychic survival.

The short story "A Scrap of Time" (1988) offers in its exposition a succinct description of the narrator's inner struggle between traumatic time, which holds experiences that do not permit representation or linear registration, and concrete, realistic time:

> I want to talk about a certain time not measured in months and years. For so long I have wanted to talk about this time, and not in the way I will talk about it now, not just about this one scrap of time. I wanted to, but I couldn't, I didn't know how. I was afraid, too, that this second time, which is measured in months and years, had buried the other time under a layer of years, that this second time had crushed the first and destroyed it within me.
>
> (Fink, 1988, p. 3)

The narrator does not fear traumatic time's triumph over concrete time, but rather the opposite, i.e. the triumph of concrete time over traumatic time and the reduction such a triumph entails.

> But no. Today, digging around in the ruins of memory, I found it fresh and untouched by forgetfulness. This time was measured not in months but in a word.
>
> (p. 3)

A deceptively circular time, as pointed out also in the context of Perec's writing, the time of trauma is not measured by linear means, and therefore what happens in it is not registered in units of time but rather in words, that is, in the registering units of the inner world.

> [...] we no longer said "in the beautiful month of May,"[1] but "after the first 'action'[2] or the second, or right before the third." We had different measures of time, we different ones, always different, always with the mark of difference [...]. We, who because of our difference were condemned once again, as we had been before in our history, we were condemned once again during this time measured not in months nor by the rising and setting of the sun, but by a word – "action", a word signifying movement, a word you would use about a novel or a play.
>
> (p. 4)

The word "action" signals the fault line dividing between the habitual rules of perception and thinking and the traumatic exile from them. The story "A Scrap of Time", however, recounts not only the first Aktion the narrator witnessed, but also the story of the collapse of one language into another:

> [...] I had left my house after eating a perfectly normal breakfast, at a table that was set in a normal way, in a room whose doors opened onto a garden veiled in morning mists, dry and golden in the rising sun. Our transformation was not yet complete; we were still living out of habit in that old time that was measured in months and years, and on that lovely peaceful morning, filled with dry, golden mists, we took the words "conscription of labor" literally [...]
>
> (p. 4)

The line the narrator draws between the old time and the new time makes a cut between the old time, in which words could be taken literally, and the new time dominated by a duplicity that transforms the spoken text into an uncanny zone. It is not only the objective world that due to duplication (manifest in the gap between the golden, misty morning and the fact that this was the morning of the first Aktion) transforms, but so do words: from now on every word conceals a meaning that is alien to its simple, familiar one. The narrator attests that on the morning of the first Aktion, she and her family were still in an "infantile state", in which they assumed that events were subject to the rules of logic. It therefore seemed possible to conduct themselves according to these rules. Thus, it was decided that the older people would disobey the Nazis' order, under the pretext that they were unfit for labor, whereas the young, for whom it would be more difficult to excuse their absence, would present themselves as required.

The infantile stage is the stage when language is not yet double, just as the text is not yet a cover story. This is the stage in which every word simply attests to its content. And yet, along this seam between the old language and the new language, the old time and the new time, she describes an interesting moment in which, without having given herself account why, she instinctively progressed from the infantile state to a state of caution when she decided to stray from the main street:

> It was then, probably at that very moment, that I suddenly progressed, instinctively, from an infantile state to a still naïve caution – instinctively, because I wasn't thinking about why I avoided the gate that led to the street and instead set off on a roundabout route [...]. Instinctively, because at that moment I still did not know that I wouldn't stand in the marketplace in front of the town hall. Perhaps I wanted to delay that moment, or perhaps I simply liked the river.
>
> (p. 15)

In the following lines, she describes how she and her sister walk along the river, as they always have, still untroubled, skipping stones across the water and dangling their legs over the riverbank. It is only when the marketplace, filled with a silent crowd, comes into view that they come to a halt:

> There was the square, thick with people as on a market day, only different, because a market-day crowd is colorful and loud, with [...] people talking and bargaining. This crowd was silent. In a way it resembled a rally – but it was different from that, too. I don't know what it was exactly. I only know that we suddenly stopped and my sister began to tremble, and then I caught the trembling [...]
>
> (p. 6)

In the attempt to characterize the silent crowd in the marketplace, she discovers, in retrospect, that although there was nothing outwardly unusual about the spectacle, she must have picked up something different, something that did not abide by the regular rules and stood out – though how she didn't have the means to tell – from everything hitherto familiar. Unlike a crowd gathered for a rally, or a crowd on any other market-day, this crowd was nothing she could put into a familiar category. It was as a result of the inability to put the sight into a familiar category that she and her sister had the paralyzing experience of uncanniness. In retrospect, she understands that at that moment her intuition preceded her conscious thinking and stopped her on time as if her "inner witness" (Amir, 2012) was recruited in order to attest to something whose existence had not yet been communicated to her conscious mind.

The two sisters then run away and sit on the slope amongst the bushes, out of breath and shaking. From where they sit they can observe their own house and the garden which looks unchanged, as well as the neighbor who has just stepped outside in order to beat the carpets. The narrator, here, puts herself and her sister in a sort of intermediate position from which both the past and the future can be observed: the regular time zone (the house, the neighbor, the slapping sounds of the carpet beater) as well as the new one (the silent crowd on the marketplace). This description of the two sisters watching the house from afar rather than offering a merely physical, concrete rendering of their situation, attests to a position of witnessing: having shifted from one territory into another enables them to see both what lies before the fault line and what awaits beyond it:

> We sat there for an hour, maybe two, I don't know, because it was then that time measured in the ordinary way stopped.
>
> (p. 16)

This blending of the new time with the old time makes it difficult to place the events along a linear narrative axis. One of the characteristics of the language of trauma is the difficulty it poses to constructing the occurrence even in retrospect. It is as if the fragmentation that crucially marks the event, comes to dominate the entire story, turns it upside down, thus preventing orderly narration: as if to say that things cannot be told "in good order" in a world in which order itself has collapsed, or as if to say that once one is thrown out from the "infantile" state of thinking, language is forever broken. The narrator, therefore, fails to narrate the story which was told to her when she returned home:

> Then we climbed down the steep slope to the river and returned to our house, where we heard what had happened in the market place, and that our cousin David had been taken, and how they took him, and what message he had left for his mother. After they were taken away, he wrote down again what he had asked people to tell her; he threw a note out of the truck and a peasant brought it to her that evening – but that happened later. [...] Only the end of the war brought us the truth about his last hours. The peasant who delivered the note did not dare to tell us what he saw, and although other people, too, muttered something about what they had seen, no one dared to believe it [...]. They went to such trouble, created so many phantoms, that only time, time measured not in months and years, opened our eyes and convinced us.
>
> (pp. 6–7)

Times in this short story mix in a manner that is not coincidental. In fact, the text enacts what the narrator discusses from the very outset: an experience of time that does not form a common, linear continuum but rather isolates and splits. In this "other" time, familiar characters act in an unfamiliar manner: the sisters who were expected to go to the square choose a roundabout route and never arrive; their cousin, with uncharacteristic eagerness (the narrator notes that he was "round-faced and chubby, not at all energetic, the sort of person who can't be pulled away from his book, who smiles 'timidly, girlishly'" – p. 7) thrusts himself forward, out of his hiding place into the line of fire; the responsible adults in the family send the young ones to the square while saving their own skins.

It seems that in the new time people become detached from their regular domain of thinking and action, and are exiled to a foreign territory in which it is no longer possible to predict anything with reference to the old terminology and habits. This ongoing deviation occurs by way of a parallel process both on the level of concrete action (the sisters taking a different route; the cousin leaving the room in which he was told to hide) as well as in the literary or textual action which shifts incessantly from the concrete description of the event to the attempt to extract a new set of meanings from it.

The story "The Garden That Floated Away" (Fink, 1988) also touches upon deviation from the concrete traumatic reality into another reality. At the beginning of the story the narrator is seated on the porch steps of her house in the afternoon, looking at the two gardens before her, the one belonging to her own home, while the other belongs to the neighbors' house. The two houses are "twin houses", and both gardens are connected, forming a single unit. A fence was never erected between them since a fence, so the residents thought, would be a foreign element.

Although a fence was not erected, another, much more foreign element now divides the fate of one garden from that of the other. Up until the point in time when this story begins, the residents of the two houses would do the garden chores at the same time. Perhaps this is why the neighbors' son announces, out of habit, that he and his sister are about to pick the russet apples. The narrator and her sister remain seated on the porch steps, while inside the house their father is talking to a woman called Mrs. Kasinska. Slowly, the vastness of the abyss gaping between the semi-detached houses and the two connected gardens becomes clear. While one house continues to live as always, the morning's only concern being that the picked russet apples must be put carefully side by side to avoid bruising them – in the twin house nothing is as it was before:

> We were sitting on the porch steps, waiting for Father to finish talking with Mrs. Kasinska and call us in. Their conversation was taking place in his office, which was dusty and unused now, though sometimes a patient still appeared in the evening under cover of darkness with a loaf of black bread in his basket as payment.
>
> (1988, p. 12)

Though they are not explicitly mentioned, between the lines are implied the hunger (a simple loaf of bread serves as payment), the persecution (patients come only under the cover of darkness; the father and Mrs. Kasinska discuss how much she will be paid for getting the girls new identity cards to save their lives), and the loss of a whole former life (the father's dusty and unused office). As they sit on the porch steps, watching the neighbors' son and his sister pick apples, the narrator overhears fragments of their conversation:

> They were saying that we had eaten up all our fruit while it was still green, and that we were right to do so, because who knows what would happen to us by winter. What they were saying was absolutely true.
>
> (p. 13)

The indifference with which the neighbor children's words are uttered – words describing facts and actions devoid of their deeper meaning, devoid of their implications, which pertain not merely to the russet apples but to matters of life and death – signals the banal version of evil to which this story serves as a stage. There is neither offensive intent nor hatred, but rather a lack of awareness on account of which the residents of the twin house can starve to death near their childhood friends and neighbors without the latter taking any note of it.

This is when the narrator begins to daydream, or perhaps hallucinate, that the neighbors' garden is sailing away:

> Wojciech's garden, the garden of our childhood friend, suddenly shuddered, swayed, began to pitch and roll, and slowly, slowly, it started to float away, like a huge green ocean liner. It sealed away slowly but steadily; the distance between us grew quickly, the garden got smaller and disappeared. It had floated away to an inaccessible distance, far beyond our reach.
>
> (p. 13)

This psychic occurrence is interrupted when her sister says to her:

> Don't squint like that. When you squint anyone can see right away that you're Jewish.
>
> As soon as she said that, everything suddenly returned to its place [...]. But who could believe in such a return? Not me.
>
> (pp. 13–14)

The state of daydreaming or hallucination into which the narrator symbolically sinks represents the growing gap not only between the fate of the narrator's family and that of their neighbors but also between that time and this time, the territory prior to the traumatic rift and the territory following it. In this context, it is interesting that what brings the narrator back to reality from her hallucination is her sister saying that her squint exposes her to danger. In other words, the inner realm is no less dangerous than the actual reality. In both of these territories, it is impossible to reside.

The common denominator of the two stories discussed thus far relates to the act of deviating from the territory of reality into another territory which serves as a position (physical or mental) from which one can observe the truth lucidly and impartially. In both stories, the narrating characters seek a point in space or time from which they may observe the changing reality. In the first story this movement takes the shape of the narrator inexplicably straying from the main road and situating herself in a hiding place from which she can observe the goings on, whereas in the second story the movement is into the territory of reverie or hallucination, which throws a clear light on the illusion that preserves the twin houses, and how it conceals a split and riven fate.

Yet the second story adds an additional layer to the first: it points to the danger not only of residing in the traumatic reality but equally of deviating from it. For while in the story "A Scrap of Time" straying from the usual route saves the narrator's life, here straying into reverie jeopardizes the narrator by exposing her identity. Survival therefore depends on the possibility of preserving an almost unbearable tension between two poles: on the one hand, it is necessary to deviate from the concrete reality in order to bear witness to it; on the other hand one must preserve a firm connection with that reality in order to survive it.

The tension between these two poles is chillingly demonstrated in the story "The Key Game" (Fink, 1988). This story, like the two previous ones, involves an attempt to sidestep reality. Here the deviation is into a "cover story". The narrative opens with a scene in which two parents are training their three-year-old son to adopt a cover story. To the child, they present the effort as a game. The mother imitates the sound of the doorbell and the child stages a scene in which he seemingly, and unsuccessfully, looks for the key. This creates time for his father to enter the pre-arranged hiding place:

> It was late, past ten o'clock. The day had long since ended, and they could have gone to sleep, but first they had to play the game that they had been playing every day for two weeks and still had not got right.
>
> (pp. 35–36)

In spite of the attempt to make it all look like a game, the father's intense anxiety and paleness, every time he steps out of his hiding place, expose that for him it is a matter of life and death. This causes the boy to freeze, staring at the closed door of the bathroom, waiting to see the father emerge at the end of the game. When, finally, the father steps out, blinking (we learn that he began blinking like this soon after the family fled their previous apartment), the parents turn to the child:

> "That's right," the woman said, "you're really doing a wonderful job, darling – and you're not little at all. You act just like a grown up, don't you? And you do know that if Mama is at work, everything will depend on you? Isn't that right? And what will you say when they ask you about your parents?"
> "Mama's at work."
> "And Papa?"
> He was silent.
> "And Papa?" the man screamed in terror.
> The child turned pale.
> "And Papa?" the man repeated more calmly.
> "He's dead," the child answered and threw himself at his father, who was standing right beside him, blinking his eyes in that funny way, but who was already long dead to the people who would really ring the bell.
>
> (pp. 37–38)

The paradox in this story is that for the child, the cover story is much more terrible than the concrete reality. To say that his father is dead is to say the worst of all, and the paradox relates to him having to testify to the worst of all so that the worst of all will not happen. Here, too, as in "A Scrap of Time", time derives from the word: the boy "gains" time while verbally staging the search, and is obliged to declare his father's death in order to "sentence" him to life. But this is not all there is to this paradox: for it is by telling the cover story that the boy testifies to the truth. The cover story, the territory of deviation, is a shocking and exact replica of what is about to take place in reality, and therefore rather than a story that covers, it is a story that reveals. In other words, the territory to which the parents deviate is not only a cover narrative but also a testimonial one. Perhaps unknowingly the parents are preparing the child for what will ensue following the knock on the door: the father will die and so will he. As in the previous stories, the characters deviate from the existing reality in order to bear witness to it, and this deviation, whose a priori purpose is to enable an escape from reality, is also what constitutes the most precise and cruel perspective on this reality.

The story "Habhila" ("nausea"; Fink, 2004)[3] demonstrates another type of deviation: deviation into the physical symptom. Nausea simultaneously expresses fusion and distancing. We tend to feel nauseous wherever there is insufficient distance between us and something, that is, in response to experiencing it, whether consciously or not, as too close. The thing that causes the nausea does not necessarily arouse objective repulsion. It may be an intense perfume piercing our nostrils, a face that pushes itself too close to ours, imagined contact with something we usually avoid. Repulsion is bound up with the collapse of distance: it comes to "repair" or restore that distance by the concrete or imagined vomiting out the intrusive object. Nausea, then, is both the result of the loss of distance, as well as what aims at rehabilitating it. It is an expression of too much closeness which instigates, or imposes, removal (Amir, 2014).

The story "Nausea" deals with the possibility of creating a distance from a traumatic object. The physical symptom, in this case, serves as testimony both to the lack of distance from the catastrophic event as well as to the need to recreate such a distance. Anna and Joseph come to visit Mira and Yan in a town at whose train station Anna was taken prisoner thirty years ago. The actual event remains vague throughout the story, apparently to Anna herself as well. Through its ambiguity, the story in fact enacts Anna's inner struggle between the obsessive need to revisit the traumatic scene and the stubborn refusal to remember it. The struggle between the compulsion to repeat and the wish to repress is manifest not only in Anna's own inner tension, but also in the tension between herself and the other characters: Mira, who does not understand Anna's failure to create a distance from the catastrophic memory; Joseph, Anna's partner, who warns Anna ("one must be cautious with memory" – p. 256) not merely against the elusiveness of memory, but also against the inundation it involves; and Yan, Mira's partner, who jokes about the traumatic events, diminishing in that way their catastrophic volume.

The story focuses on the attempt to situate the catastrophic events in the current present. When they arrive at Mira and Yan's house and meet a couple of middle-aged neighbors, Yan recounts how in the first years after the war, whenever they met someone over forty, the question of what he or she had done at that time would come up. Further on, Mira mentions that they have good relations with their neighbors. It is implicitly clear that good neighborly relations of this kind can only be based on ignoring the past and leaving unasked the abysmal question of what these neighbors had done at the time.

The characters in this story exhibit different levels of distancing from the traumatic memory, and different modes of situating it in the present. Anna is alone in being unable either to take a distance or to forget, the only one who cannot move forward. She is not interested in seeing the town nor is she willing to cooperate with any attempt to redeem the horror. She has come in order to meet that horror, to return to where it took place. The only deviation she allows herself takes the form of a state of bodily disorientation, a state of nausea that symbolically situates her between the inability to swallow her memories and the inability to spit them out.

At some point Joseph says to Anna:

> You must get rid of it, my dear, but I warn you: expect disappointment, you will not find 'your' train station.
>
> (p. 256)

Joseph highlights the essence of the problem of memory: since Anna cannot return to the memory, she cannot get rid of it either. The story presents the traumatic event as being doomed to stay stuck or imprisoned between stomach and mouth, impossible to either digest or discharge, not even through speech ("Anna did not want to speak about the subject, she wanted only to see" – p. 254). Nausea, much like daydreaming, the cover story and the route bypassing the marketplace, is a deviation that constitutes the position of the witness. This particular position of the witness, however, belongs to the psychotic mode which enables neither a connection to the experience nor an observant, reflective distancing from it.

The story "Description of a Morning" (Fink, 1997) expands this theatre which is performed this time on a stage whose only set is a crack in the wall of an attic where a woman and a man are hiding. The crack is their only window to the world, and the man stays fixed to it while incessantly reporting what is happening outside to the woman who is lying down, inactive and motionless. The reason for his relentless chatter (practicing Latin, obsessively memorizing names of pupils in his former class and so on) is his fear that if he were to fall silent, unbearable thoughts would invade his consciousness. For the same reason he also forbids his wife to think:

Woman: I can't. I don't want to. I can't bear this anymore.
Man: So think of something else.

Woman: I just want to sit in silence.
Man: Silence is our enemy. I've explained that hundreds of times.
(p. 85)

Gradually it becomes clear that the traumatic memory, the right to which she is fighting for while he struggles to make her forget, is the memory of their little daughter who was shot to death before their eyes:

Woman: Always the same dream. I don't dream of anyone else. Not my parents, not your brother Elek, not Aunt Regina and her son. Nobody. How did it happen, Artur? If I hadn't let go of her hand ... She saw a cat. "Mama, a little cat! On the wall, a little cat!" She said that, and then she was gone. Artur, do you remember how it happened? Because I don't ... I don't remember anything.
(p. 90)

When the man finally surrenders to his wife's wish and together with her reconstructs the words the German soldier said at the moment he shot the little girl, the woman understands that had the child stayed with them, they would not have been able to escape; that the death of their child was the sacrifice that enabled their survival:

Woman: And if he hadn't killed her, if she had gone on with us, with the rest of us? You and I wouldn't have been able to get away. She was small, she couldn't run fast. And she didn't understand ... Isn't it true that if she had gone with us, we wouldn't have been able to get away?
(p. 95)

This understanding seems to touch on the most unbearable experience. The next day, when the man wakes up, he discovers that his wife is gone. Fink's enigmatic style leaves us the option to understand this either as the woman's literal disappearance or her death. By dying (or by escaping from the attic which would be tantamount to suicide), the woman can be seen to patch together the fragmented narrative: in effect she puts herself to death as she would indeed have died had she stayed with her child. The most severe trauma is not merely the event itself, but the fragmentation the subject must maintain in order not to meet what a possible narrative sequence might expose. The woman in this story chooses to forego the deviation that was imposed (and enabled) by her daughter's death and reverts to the original scenario, in which she does not let go of the girl's hand but rather joins her. In fact, it is through her death that she reclaims her life as a sequence, as a whole.

With its minimalist dialogue, this story unfolds the core of the conflict that defines the position of the witness and the very act of testimony. Of the two characters, the woman is the one who insists on bearing witness. For her the only possibility is to be a full witness, that is, to remember, so when her husband prevents her from doing so he prevents her from being. He, by contrast, rejects both the act of bearing witness as well as the position of the witness. He is willing to bear witness to what was prior to the catastrophic event; he is even ready to create a new reality and bear witness to it through a play he writes, but he refuses to bear witness to the traumatic rift of his daughter's death. His incessant talk, therefore, is not a manifestation of thought but an attack on thinking:

Woman: I just want to sit in silence.
Man: Words – and I've said this a hundred times – are our salvation.
(p. 85)

What gradually becomes clear (connecting between the events in this story and the nausea of the previous story), is that it is neither possible to cover up nor to reveal the traumatic memory and stay alive. The wife's position of the witness – a position which allows her neither to forget nor to take a distance – sentences her to death. However, the husband's hollow position of the witness does not enable life either, converting it into a mechanical mode of "staying alive".

The protagonists of this story are trapped between two forms of death: the death caused by the link to the traumatic memory, and the death caused by dissociating from it. The attic constitutes a zone of deviation located in between internal and external, past and future. This is an exterritorial and extemporal zone, situated both outside of space and outside of time (the man attests to this when he fails to figure out what day it is), and the two of them are confined in this zone, each taking their separate/complementary role: the man looking out exclusively, while the woman's gaze is directed only into herself. Neither of these polarities bears a chance. The only chance of retaining psychic life might lie in simultaneously holding the two positions and thus uniting the internal and the external gaze, the past and the present, the capacity to remember and the capacity to forget.

In the story "Traces" (Fink, 1988), the last to be discussed here, the narrator faces a photograph of the last ghetto in which she and her family stayed. She cannot reconstruct the personal circumstances in which the photograph was taken: instead she observes it in the "third person" (also literally using the third person when describing it) without connecting to the experience:

> Yes, of course she recognizes it. Why shouldn't she? That was their last ghetto. [...] Of course she is amazed. How did they survive there? Such ... such, well, it's hard to express. But in those days no one was surprised at anything.
>
> (p. 135)

The position of the "external observer" puts a distance between herself and the experience. She does not ask how she herself survived ("how did I", "how did we"), but rather "How did **they** survive there", as if she were considering a historical document whose meaning eludes her. Soon enough, however, the excessive distance switches into a lack of even the most minimal distance required to enable observation:

> She pushes the photograph away. "I prefer not to be reminded ..."
>
> (p. 136)

A moment later she picks up the photograph again:

> Again she reaches for the photograph, raises it to her nearsighted eyes, looks at it for a long time, and says, "You can still see the traces of footprints." And a moment later, "That's very strange. That's the direction they walked in." [...] She looks at the footprints, the snow, and then stalls once again. "I wonder who photographed it? And when? Probably right afterwards: the footprints are clear here, but when they shot them in the afternoon it was snowing again."
>
> (p. 136)

It is only through the narrator's rather concrete wonder regarding the survival of the traces of those who were shot that we are exposed to the catastrophe to which she testifies. Exposure, here, is not via amplification but rather via attenuation. Through the marginal reference to the traces, we find ourselves tracing the story of the children whose parents hid them in the attic of the Judenrat, and who were caught and then murdered. The text's shifting between distant observation and getting drawn into the catastrophe is an extreme yet imperceptible movement. In the same breath, she pushes the photograph away and also asks that everything she says will be preserved forever. In a single moment she shifts from alienated puzzlement at the physical traces in the snow, to her wish that the erased traces of the children's story be captured forever in the narrative she inscribes on the white paper:

> "I prefer not to remember ..." But suddenly she changes her mind and asks that what she is going to say be written down and preserved forever, because she wants a trace to remain.
>
> (p. 136)

Perhaps she understands at this moment that leaving a trace on behalf of the children is the only way for her to stay alive, not only as the sole physical survivor but also as a full witness. What is fascinating here is the transformation in the narrator's position of the witness. At the beginning of the story, she looks at the photograph as a stranger. Soon she notices the traces in the snow, and this transports her at once into the photograph. From that moment onwards she is no longer a bystander. She may well have been one of these children, having miraculously survived. Her testimony moves therefore from a most remote position (reminding us of Perec's position of the witness at the beginning of his book: "I am not the hero of my tale, nor am I exactly its bard" – p. 4) to one that is extremely close, in which the witness is not only an observer but also the protagonist of the scene.

The story leads her and the reader through all these different points of view: the alienated perspective that refuses to believe; that of the bystander; and finally, the point of view of the one who was present at the very heart of the catastrophic event itself. One may understand the narrator's transformation as one which shifts from the psychotic inability to form any connection with the experience to being metonymically drawn into it – to the metaphoric mode of witnessing, which does not alienate itself from the story or collapse into it, but rather becomes its owner.

Notes

1 In reference to Heinrich Heine's poem, "Im Wunderschöne Monat Mai".
2 Aktion.
3 This story does not appear in the collections of short stories translated to English: *A Scrap of Time* (1988) and *Traces* (1997). The quotes from the story are freely translated from the Hebrew version that appears in *Kol HaSipurim* (2004) [Collected stories].

References

Amir, D. (2012). The inner witness. *International Journal of Psycho-Analysis*, 93, 879–896.
Amir, D. (2014). *Cleft tongue*. New York and London: Karnac Books.
Fink, I. (1988). *A scrap of time: And other stories*. (trans: M. Levine and F. Prose). London: Peter Owen Publishers.
Fink, I. (1997). *Traces: Stories*. (trans: P. Boehm and F. Prose). New York: Henry Holt and Company.
Fink, I. (2004). *Kol HaSipurim*. Tel Aviv, Israel: Am Oved Publishers.
Perec, G. ([1975] 2010). *W or the memory of childhood*. (trans: D. Bellos). Boston, MA: D. R. Godine.

Chapter 7

From the collapse of signifiers to the reconstruction of language

Robert Antelme's *The Human Race*[1]

Robert Antelme, a member of a French Resistance group headed by Francois Mitterrand, was arrested by the Gestapo in June 1944, sent to Buchenwald, then to a work camp in Germany where he almost died. This moving memoir, his only book, is dedicated to the task of tracing the outline of the "human" from the perspective of both victim and witness. Its close observation of language's most subtle nuances, in an uncompromising effort to represent the event in terms of the event rather than in those of the observer, makes its reading uncommonly demanding. This demand constitutes itself the gravest and most exposed self-testimony, one in which Antelme constantly warns against slipping into "comfortable" categories and against a possible escape into the saturated state of the "gratified" conscience. Whether they concern the executioners or their victims, his descriptions are marked by the same gentle restlessness which turns its penetrating gaze upon the observer no less than upon the object of observation.

Primo Levi (1979), describing a recurrent dream about Auschwitz, points at it in one word:

> A single word, not imperious, but brief and subdued. It is the dawn command of Auschwitz, a foreign word, feared and expected: get up, "Wstawach".
>
> (p. 380)

Antelme, too, points at a word that became etched in his memory: "Fertig!" – "that's it!" (Antelme, [1957] 1992, p. 18). Sometimes, as Ida Fink wrote (1988), time is measured by a word. It is not just a word that holds the difference between the before and the after, the pre-traumatic and the traumatic. Somehow this word is so powerful exactly because it is quoted and not told – i.e. by its being directed straight at the reader, a call one cannot ignore, a rupture in the continuous language or a moment when regular language collapses into the language of trauma. Unlike the other words, it is uttered in its original language, with its original sound, thus becoming signifier and signified at one and the same time, something that by pointing at the rupture constitutes the very rupture itself. And so the collapse signaled by Levi's "Wstawac!" ("Get up!"), much like Antelme's "Fertig!" ("That's it!"), is related to the unconscious call (which is nevertheless enfolded in memory by way of the word's exact sound) to wake up to the nightmare which tore the world apart.

> A deep voice, well modulated, almost melancholy. [...] It is an SS man who is talking. In that sober tone he calls the head of the block, a Kapo, or some other staff member; but it is indeed a prisoner whom he is addressing. We had heard it often, that voice, coming over the barracks loudspeaker. It would spread over the entire camp: "Kapos ... Kapos," with a deep *a*. That was the word that recurred most often. At the beginning, it had appeared mysterious. In reality, that voice and that word manifested the whole organization. Calm and composed, the voice directed everything. Between the voice and the regime imposed by the SS it seemed at first impossible to make any connection.
>
> (Antelme, [1957] 1992, p. 19)

The horror resides not just in the abominations themselves: it inheres in the gaping abyss between the meaning of these acts and the calm and serenity with which they are carried out; in the fact that death can be managed like this: a deep, long-stretched *a*, in a pleasant voice, at ease. The voice fills barracks and camp, allowing a softness to seep in along with cruelty, to the point that the distinction between what constitutes death and what constitutes life becomes blurred.

Antelme notices that in the seemingly random exchanges between the prisoners while they do their forced labor, they often mention things they owned in the past, especially the food they so badly lack now:

> Each of us will already be with somebody else in a little while. He'll explain how his mother makes custard, because he needs to talk about

> custard and milk and bread. [...] We'll invite each other over to dinner, because by inviting each other we can picture still more meat, more bread. And then, if tonight there are seconds of soup, this guy who's invited his buddy to come to dinner along with his wife may elbow him out of the way.
>
> (ibid., p. 44)

Not only does speech turn from a mode of communication into a mode of survival, placing the other, the random listener, as a means rather than as a target for that talk, but words from being signifiers become signifieds: talk about bread takes the place of the bread; the invitation to a meal stretches the limits of the concrete stomach by increasing the number of imaginary guests. In the traumatized domain of language, the symbolic gradually collapses into the excess of real suffering.

> It may be language that deceives us; it's the same back there as it is here; we use the same words, pronounce the same names. So we begin to worship that language, since it has become the ultimate thing that we possess in common. Sometimes when I am in the neighborhood of a German I speak French with special attentiveness, in a way I don't ordinarily speak it back home; I construct sentences better, I use all sorts of elisions, with as much care, as much pleasure as if I were putting together a song. With German nearby, our tongue rings, I see it shape itself as I speak it. I bring it to a halt, I make it swell in the air anew, do what I wish with it; it's mine. [...] Our language doesn't make the SS laugh; it merely confirms our condition. In a low voice, in a loud voice, even in silence, it's always the same, inviolable. They can do a great deal but they can't teach us another language which would be the language of the prisoner. [...] Though we become unrecognizable to our kin, this certainty shall always remain to us: of yet employing this babble of our youth and of our old age which is the permanent and ultimate form of our independence and identity.
>
> (pp. 45–46)

Language is the stage for Antelme's most relentless struggle for vividness, now radically tested by the stagnation of the traumatic reality. He points at it as the one shelter, the one certainty, the one inviolable signifier of identity, the bridge between the traumatic "here" and home's "there".

How immune is language to catastrophe? One may understand what Antelme describes here as his holding on to language as to his own "lyrical dimension"[2] integrating the constant and the ever-becoming aspects of identity (Amir, 2016). On the one hand, language is in charge of the aspect of ongoingness, of the continuity between "here" and "there": "it's always the same, inviolable" (ibid.). On the other hand, however, Antelme uses language as a creative substrate onto which he fashions himself as he wishes, and in that sense he appropriates language, differently each time, right in the face of the SS officer, that is to say, right in the face of the catastrophic present.

One might have expected that the catastrophic reality would cause language to collapse either towards the "continuous pole" (Amir, 2016), the pole of sameness (or facelessness) which preserves its common elements at the cost of its singularity, or alternatively to collapse towards the "emergent pole" (Amir, 2016) of mere singularity, entailing autistic or psychotic encapsulation at the cost of communication (Amir, 2014). But Antelme insists exactly on the integration of these two poles as what characterizes his language of survival, and this enables him to preserve both the stable form of his identity as well as the flexibility needed for survival especially amid the catastrophe.

One of the most interesting moments in this context of identity survival occurs when he is told to sweep a room, in which there is a German girl and behind her "a solid block of German males" (Antelme, [1957] 1992, p. 50). Surprisingly, he turns this sweeping into a sophisticated game of visibility and invisibility:

> Then I went after another piece of paper, next to another shoe. The German moved his foot the way you brush a fly away from your forehead when you're asleep, without waking up. I was something roaming in their sleep. [...] they didn't see me, but their bodies moved; to the extent that I didn't exist for them, they were submissive. But the girl was wide awake. She had been following my performance; she knew I was playing a game; she knew I was going after those scraps of paper only in order to crowd those godlike figures and make them move their feet. She couldn't denounce me for that would have required an explanation since they wouldn't have understood right away; and so she would have ended up showing that she wasn't as mighty as they were, since she had noticed me. She would have brought me on stage,

> rendered me visible, and they would have been obliged to talk to me, to formulate words for me, in order to make me completely invisible again, in order to get rid of me.
>
> (Antelme, [1957] 1992, pp. 50–51)

It is not by means of the actions that Antelme maps out what's going on but rather by means of what these actions negate: the existence of the prisoner as a subject. The Germans' unconscious moving of their feet as he is picking up scraps of paper from below them seem to be part of a comprehensive choreography that comes to nullify his existence as an-other. They are asleep in his presence, that is to say: they do not experience him as a human being whose presence demands their attention. The girl, by contrast, is awake. Aware of his presence as a subject, her peace of mind is disturbed. By sending him out of the room she, in fact, acknowledges him more than do the men who let him be, and thus reveals her weakness: she identifies him as a human subject and hence cannot ignore him. This map Antelme sketches not only depicts the general rules of the "game" of the camp, but also shows what he himself brings into play in order to avoid being erased in the course of this game: his capacity to recognize the rules of their language as well as its zones of transgression. His affirmation as a subject in this episode is not related merely to the girl's telling him to get out of the room, but even more so to his own sense of the meaning of his being told to leave and the way this paradoxically made him "be in".

> The SS man's stare, his behavior towards us – which never varied – meant that for him no difference existed between one prisoner's face and another's. When we were at roll call, five abreast, the SS man had to be able to count five heads in each column. [...] A face was distinguishable only by some additional object – eye glasses for example, which in this sense were a calamity. And if someone had to *stay* distinguishable, the Kapos, so as not to lose him, would draw a red circle and a white circle on the back of his striped jacket. Furthermore, no one, by means of his face, was to express to the SS anything that might have been the beginning of a dialogue and that might have been able to bring into being upon the SS man's face anything else than the permanent and impartial negation reserved for everyone. Thus, as a face was not only useless but also, in spite of itself, rather dangerous, in our relations with the SS we reached the point where we made an

> effort to negate our faces ourselves, an effort which perfectly matched the negation practiced by the SS. Denied, double denied [...] our face had, for us, finally become absent from our life.
>
> (Antelme, [1957] 1992, pp. 51–52)

Here, as in the previous paragraph, Antelme's bearing witness to the "language rules" of the game, i.e. to the double role of this negation, being the simultaneous outcome of German oppression and the only way to escape that very oppression – turns out to become his private "negation of the negation".

> That particular Sunday I look at length at my face in the mirror. It was neither beautiful nor ugly; it was dazzling. It had accompanied me here, here it was on the loose. It was without employment now, but it was still itself, the machine for expression. Next to it an SS mug was nothing. And the face of the guy who when his turn came was going to look at himself in it remained reduced to the state determined by the SS. Only the one in the mirror was distinct. It alone signified something that couldn't be accepted here. This piece of glass opened out upon a mirage. We weren't that way here. We were only that way all alone in the mirror.
>
> (p. 52)

Antelme's gaze as it captures his own face – not his face as his friends in the concentration camp or the SS officers see it, but his face as it is reflected only to him, and only in his own eyes – constitutes a moment in which he is present as an indelible subject; a subject whose gaze still identifies, in the image reflected by the mirror, his inalienable identity. But this moment of recognition also brings along the danger that accompanies it:

> However, even if I hadn't had to pass the mirror on to somebody else, I would have let it go, because I was already contaminating the face in it. It was getting old; it was going to model itself on the standard face around here, sagging, wretched, like a pair of hands one stares at hollowed-eyed.
>
> (p. 53)

This ambiguity of his reflection is related to the ambiguity of his singular identity, being both his source of power and the most serious threat he might face. This is why he simultaneously clings to it (keeping his face very close to the mirror) and negates it (contaminating the face in the mirror until its singularity is erased).

> There are guys who will perhaps be respected back home but who, for us, have become as horrifying as our worst enemies there – even more horrifying. And there are also those we didn't expect anything from, guys whose lives back home were altogether undistinguished, but who have shown themselves heroes here. [...] The SS who view us all as one and the same cannot [...] prevent us from choosing. On the contrary: here the need to choose is constant and immeasurably greater. The more transformed we become, the farther we retreat from back home, the more the SS believe us reduced to the indistinctness and to the irresponsibility [...] – the more distinctions our community does in fact contain, and the stricter those distinctions are. The inhabitant of the camps is not the abolition of these differences; on the contrary, he is their effective realization.
>
> (p. 88)

Identity, on the one hand, may undermine physical survival because a person can easily find himself exposed by certain characteristics that make him stand out in the faceless mass, not least the outlines of his personality which might form an obstacle given the demand to blend in. Holding on to identity and singularity is, however, at the same time the one way of being saved. It is exactly in the face of the Nazi regime's demand to erase all differences between the camp prisoners, thus to erase their personality as well as humanity, that these differences get reinstated with a vengeance. These differences embody their ineradicable humanity. This is why the question who takes the role of the hero and who the role of the traitor is less important than the distinction itself between heroes and traitors, which serves as a confirmation of the fact that human singularity endures even here.

Maintaining singularity is in part related to the freedom to crack the hermetic-excessive bloc of suffering by generating a surprising movement:

> We believe that what we'd like is to be able to kill this SS man. But, if we think about it a little, we see that we are mistaken. It isn't so simple. What we would like is to start by turning him upside down, to fix

> him with his feet in the air. And then to laugh and laugh. Since we are men, since we are human beings, we'd also like to play a little. We'd quickly get tired of it; but that's it, that's what we'd like: his head down, his feet in the air. That's what we would like to do to the gods.
> (p. 79)

Of special interest here is Antelme's choice to turn the SS man upside down rather than kill him. Killing means erasing the other by means of turning into that other in all his cruelty. But turning that other upside down is tantamount to restoring order: a dent is made in the frozen, measureless present of the camp through the most distinctive, yet the most unpredictable, of human gestures: humor.

> Were we to go and find an SS and show Jacques to him, to him we could say: "Have a look, you have turned him into this rotten, yellowish creature. You have succeeded in making him what you think he is by nature: waste, offal. Well, we can tell you this, which by all rights would flatten you for good if 'error' could kill: you have enabled him to make of himself the strongest, the most complete of men, the surest of his powers, of the resources of his conscience, of the scope of his actions. [...] With Jacques, you never won. You wanted him to steal. He didn't steal. You wanted him to kiss the capos' asses in order to eat. He wouldn't do it. You wanted him to laugh in order to look good when a *Meister* was beating some guy up. He didn't laugh. Most of all you wanted him to doubt whether any cause was worth his rotting away like this. He didn't doubt. You get your rocks off looking at this wasted wreck that stands before you; but you're the one who's been fucked all the way up and down. We show you nothing but boils, sores, gray heads, leprosy; and that's what you believe in, the leprosy. You sink deeper and deeper."
> (pp. 88–89)

These words bear out concretely how the gods of the SS are upended, their heads down and their feet in the air. The liberating power of human thought is put on display when Antelme shows how thinking can overturn the ostensible state of affairs, crown the losers as the winners, and the winners as forsaken and deluded. If one can understand the situation differently, then it becomes bearable. If one can find the triumph concealed behind what would seem total collapse, how the power of the spirit can be revealed exactly in the body's defeat, then what has so far been experienced as an arbitrary and senseless attack on humanity transforms into the very melting pot of this humanity. This is the only possible triumph: to liberate the spirit from bodily ravage; to set free the individual's singular identity from the oblique mass of identical actions; to extricate the very ability to choose, out of the traumatic excess of the annulled, the freedom of movement. This is the struggle for the inner function of the witness: the struggle for the freedom to escape the excess of helplessness into the position of an observer who extracts meaning from it.

> We passed the procession as we were coming back from the factory. Three men: two guys to carry the dead man, and the sentry. One more and it would have been a ceremony. The SS wouldn't have permitted it. The dead mustn't be allowed to serve as a symbol for us. Here, where there is no crematorium, our dead must disappear nevertheless. Like our sleeping, like our pissing, our natural death is tolerated, but no trace of it may be left behind, either in memory or in space. There must be no way of situating the place where a dead man lies.
>
> (p. 92)

The negation of humanity reaches its peak with the negation of death. If the dead person's grave cannot be found then his absence remains unmarked, not as if he died but as though he had never lived. The philosopher Adi Ophir in his book *The Order of Evil* (2005) claims that losing one's name means losing one's ability to leave traces to one's disappearance. He does not refer to the concrete calling of the victims by their proper or family names, but to the perpetrators' acts, which sophisticatedly erase not just the victims themselves – but also the traces of their disappearance: not their lives but the very recognition of their ever being alive.

> There are moments when you could kill yourself just in order that the SS fetch up against this limit as it confronts the impassive object you'd have become, the dead body that has turned its back on them, that doesn't give a shit about their law. The dead man will at once be stronger than they are, just as are trees and clouds and cows, which we call things and incessantly envy. [...] The dead man no longer offers them a handle. Let them savage his face, let them hack his body to

> bits, the dead man's very impassiveness, his complete inertness, will counter all the blows they strike at him.
>
> (Antelme [1957] 1992, pp. 93–94)

Using his capacity to transgress the limits of helplessness by means of the power of thinking, Antelme upends the situation here and again: the dead person, the ultimate victim and victory of SS rule, now enacts the greatest revolt against his oppressors, turning his back at them, escaping their control.

> The more our condition as men is contested by the SS, the more likely our chances of being confirmed as such. The real risk we run is that of starting to hate another guy out of envy, of being betrayed by our longings, of abandoning others. From such risks no one can be relieved.
>
> (p. 96)

The same inversion occurs here, too: The further the SS pushes the camp inmates to act inhumanly, the further their humanity stands proven. Envy, craving, betrayal, rather than testifying to the absence of humanity express humanity in the fullest sense. Again, Antelme puts the SS upside down: If the dead person, the ultimate victim, is no other than the ultimate rebel, and if what seems the absolute surrender of humanity in fact prompts the human being to display humanity at its fullest, then the hierarchy on which the catastrophic present is constructed is nothing but a fictive hierarchy occluding the truth which is its total opposite.

However, the struggle to extract meaning from what seems the absolute loss of meaning is not easy. For the circular reality of catastrophe produces an empty, hollow syntax which far from yielding discursivity that cross-fertilizes, repeats the same formulae articulating the unchanging outlines of the present:

> We linger for a moment, sitting on the rail.
> "What's new?" one of the Frenchmen asks.
> "Nothing," replies the other.
> The one who asked the question hadn't figured there was anything new. There hasn't been anything new since we got here, on the first of October. But we have asked the question every morning. The guy who's asking it now is not in a position to answer it for

> himself; all he can know is what he sees, and that's always the same thing: the bread in the morning, the factory, the latrines. Since he's been locked up everything that isn't bread or factory has been hidden from him.
>
> "Nothing," the other guy answered. He's in the same situation as the guy who asked, but he didn't say "I don't know." "Nothing" is what he said, even though he doesn't know whether there is anything new. [...]
>
> "You think it's going to be a long time?" the questioner inquires.
>
> "I don't think so."
>
> That makes the first guy feel all right. All it takes is that the other guys not be too taciturn, not reply "I don't know." Provided they stay in this hazy area, provided they don't take it into their head to ask "How do you know?" they will reassure each other. Each brings what the other awaits, like a brother, like a mother: someone other than yourself and who's not threatening, who'll bother to reply.
>
> (pp. 102–103)

This quasi-conversation can exist so long as no one abandons the rules of the game, the rules that ensure that nothing new is said, that no one will insist on validity or truth ("How do you know?"), that no words will be said other than those that serve their fixed function, namely, to allow the conversation to go on in all its sterility. Here, the other is not fully other: he is only other in so far as his physical location (outside the self) makes it possible to engage him in a pseudo-conversation which fills the empty spaces of thinking much like the straw blankets fill the holes in which the prisoners sleep.

Christmas arrives into this frozen, circular present. A single marker of time arises in this traumatic eternity located outside any form of human periodization:

> The siren sounded at four o'clock, and we left the factory. It wasn't snowing anymore, the sky had cleared, and there was even a little sun on the woods. We arrived in front of the church and let them count us. We waited; we still had to get there, to the pallets and to Christmas Day. [...] I'm going out they are saying back home; and they go down the stairway, they're outside. "I'm going to sit down," they say; "we'll eat together," they say; and they do sit down, they do eat. "I," they say, and right away it's bread, or a bed, or the street for them. Here, all we

> can say is "I'm going to the latrine." Here that's what probably corresponds most closely to what's ordinarily called liberty back there.
>
> (p. 104)

By its very nature, language is grounded in categories of space and time and in a causal hierarchy. But in the reality of the camp time is cyclic, the space necessary for mobility has been canceled and causality is arbitrary. And so words like "I" and "go" which in the past were signifiers with concrete signifieds, stay adrift in the mouth's cavity like stray satellites. Language is ostensibly the same as always, obeying the same syntactic rules, featuring a distinct subject and object and tenses. All of these, however, are an illusion once the signified "camp" enters. There is no "I" that can serve as "subject" because the individual no longer owns his actions or has the freedom to choose whether to move or to stand still; there's no movement-affording space and no verb, therefore, can bear any meaning. And more than anything, there is no difference whatsoever between past, present and future because everything that happens is wholly subject to an ongoing, frozen present without a beginning or an end.

> I forget, every day I forget a little more; one gets farther away, one drifts. I don't hear anything anymore; [...] Knowing is all I have left. Knowing that M has a voice, the voice I know she has. Knowing that her face opens up, that she laughs the laugh I know she has. Knowing like a man who's deaf and blind. And that I am the only one here who knows that. That slowly M's very face may disappear, and then I'll really be like a blind man. But they can disguise me still more, they can do the impossible to make me barely distinguishable from somebody else, even so I'll still know that until the very end.
>
> (p. 108)

It is not only for his specific memories that Antelme is struggling here but for keeping memory itself as a territory that is not expropriated. The knowledge he describes, "knowing like a man who's deaf and blind", is one that bears no relation to the external reality, one that has been deposited inside where it is kept safe in the mere consciousness of the owner of these recollections. The possibility of "Knowing that M. has a voice, the voice I know she has" claims to hold on to the singularity of M.'s voice, and thereby also to his own singularity ("And that I am the only one here who knows that").

The greatest fear, the greatest horror is of losing one's claim to a singular identity, of losing the ownership of one's memories and narrative:

> At that point each one had become a figure in a story. The person who, yet a free man, had while chatting heard the church tower bell strike half-past four, and then had heard the same bell strike five o'clock with handcuffs on his wrists. The person who didn't show up that evening. The person who'd been nailed between two sentences. He was filling the whole house now.
>
> (p. 109)

The transition from "there" to "here" consists of an interrupted movement ("The person who'd been nailed between two sentences"). As soon as this transition occurs, no simple continuity between past and present is possible anymore, much like the movement from present to future, too, will no longer be simple.

> [...] she was praying for him as though he had some horrible disease. She didn't know that her prayer was for a stranger.
>
> (p. 109)

Had he contracted a terrible disease, his death would still have been part of the predictable continuity of life and death. But the place to which he has been exiled entertains no ongoing relation with life as it was before. He will in fact not be able to return from this place: not because he cannot survive it but because the man he once was no longer exists.

> I was alone, between the wall of the church and the SS barracks; urine steamed; I was alive. It had to be believed. Once again I looked up at the sky. I wondered if perhaps I was the only one to be looking up into the night this way. Beneath the emptiness, in the steam of the urine, amidst the dread, this was happiness. And it is doubtless thus that I must say that that night was beautiful.
>
> (p. 111)

The moments when Antelme shifts from the position of the victim to the position of the witness are indeed those in which he manages to preserve or to consolidate a consciousness, one that maintains at least certain continuity with the person who he was before the breach. The steam that the frozen ground of the urinal sends back up to him testifies to his being alive; the same is true for the beauty that is returned to him from the night into which he casts his gaze.

But there are many other moments when language and thinking are under dismaying attack:

> Degradation and flabbiness of language. Mouths whence nothing any longer ever came that was ordered, or strong enough to last. A weakly woven cloth fraying to bits. Sentences succeeded one another, contradicted one another, expressed a kind of belched up wretchedness; a bile of words. They were all jumbled together: the son of a bitch who'd done it, the wife left on her own, food, drink, the old lady's tears, the fuck-in-the-ass, and so on; the same mouth could say it all, one thing after the other. It came forth all by itself; the gut would empty. It only stopped at night. Hell must be like that, a place where everything that's said, everything that's expressed, comes forth equalized with everything else, homogenized, like a drunkard's puke.
>
> (p. 135)

Hell is the moment when language, usually in charge of distinctions and differentiations, turns into a limpid mass into which all definition bleeds and blends. This is the moment when speech stops testifying to the symbolic order and turns into an attack of diarrhea, an act of vomiting, a collapse into the Real. This is when words come to have the durability and status of body secretions.

> Fists clenched, all I squeeze is emptiness; I can feel the bones in my hands. I close my jaws, again nothing there but bone, nothing to grind, nothing that yields, not the thinnest grape-skin to put between them. I chew, I chew, but the self, the self's not chewable. I'm the chewer, something to be chewn on, something to be eaten, where does it exist? [...] Can it be possible that there is really nothing?
>
> (pp. 137–138)

In the traumatic realm of the Real there's no distinction between the one who eats and the food eaten, between the hungry and hunger. The excess of starvation cannot be contained or transformed by language (therefore the excessiveness of the mode of witnessing in this specific paragraph, which reminds us in a way of Ka-Tzetnik's style). It perforates the container's walls. This juncture at which the container of language disintegrates in the face of the excess of suffering appears frequently in Antelme's account:

> Francis wanted to talk about the sea. I resisted. Language acted like a sorcery. When your body was rotting, *the sea, water, sunshine* could make you suffocate. With these words, as with M's name, you were in danger of not wanting to take another step, not wanting to get up again. And you'd put off the moment for talking about them, you'd keep that moment in reserve, as a last resort. I knew that Francis, who was skinny and ugly like me, could hallucinate, and could make me hallucinate, with a few words. We had to defer that. So as to be able to be our own sorcerer, at that later time when we'd no longer be able to expect anything from either our bodies or our wills; when we'd be sure that we'd never see the sea again. But so long as the future was possible, we had to keep quiet.
>
> (p. 162)

This is a descent down the scale of secondary processes of thinking; a process of negative transformation in which words turn from signifiers into signifieds. Words like "sea" or "sun" transform into hallucinations of sea and sun. A new territory emerges which, constituting neither thinking nor the body, is a hybrid between them. A word stops being an expression of "thought about the body" (whether the world's body or the body of flesh and blood) and transforms into a body in itself, while the actual body transforms into absence.

One of the most terrifying illustrations of such absence is Antelme's visit to K. at the infirmary, shortly before the latter's death:

> I moved away from the bed, Several times I turned around, hoping each time that the face I knew would appear; but I couldn't find even so much as its nose. [...] Now the name remained: K. [...] Yet I hadn't been able to say, "This is K." when I was looking at him in the *Revier*. Death itself contains no greater mystery. K. was going to die that night. Which meant that he wasn't dead yet; that we'd have to wait

> before declaring dead the man I'd known, of whom I still had a picture in my head, of whom his friend had a still older picture; we had to wait till this man here, whom neither of us knew, was dead. That had happened while K. was alive; it was the living K. in whom I hadn't found anybody. Because I no longer found the man I'd known, and because he didn't recognize me, I'd had doubts about myself for a minute. It was to reassure myself that I was still me that I'd looked at other guys [...]. Just as the stable faces of the other guys had reassured me, so, in death, the dead K. was going to reassure, restoring this man's oneness. Yet it would remain true that between the man I'd known and the dead K., whom we would all know, this nothingness had existed.
>
> (pp. 172–173)

This halfway state when a person is no longer himself, i.e. he who is at one with his name and identity, and yet is not dead, is the closest to the uncanny. This is a "nothingness" relative to which even death is "something". "The dead K." will soon be a recognized entity, related both to his past and to the future he might have had. But the dying K., K. the *Muselmann*, has no biographical continuity with K. the man and therefore no history. This is a body whose very existence forms an attack on any attempt to maintain a flow or to constitute a narrative. Hence Antelme's own continuity is under attack each time he looks at K. In contrast with the stable faces of the others, K. embodies the conversion from one state (body, firm) to another (empty, absence). As such his presence undermines the observer's ability to maintain his own stability.

> Having yielded to this vice of believing anything possible, each could have risked drowning, as a result of some word or other from the past, a word that would have swollen and swollen in size and finally become a millstone hung around his neck. Then his eyes would have opened upon this afternoon, this one here [...]. And the time represented by the war would have suddenly frozen within this afternoon that continued to darken and dissolve. And he would have rediscovered hunger, true hunger.
>
> (p. 191)

Antelme deludes himself that he has the ability (associated with the symbolic order) to use language manipulatively, to produce a back-and-forth movement by means of words. All of a sudden, however, thinking breaks down as one word grows heavier and heavier until it blocks the entire inner space.

In his essay "The Uncanny" (1955 [1919]) Freud writes that a sense of the uncanny arises wherever the boundary between reality and imagination grows vague, when something we considered fantastic appears real, or when the symbol absorbs the full function and meaning of the thing symbolized. The moment a word turns into a millstone is indeed a moment in which the symbol loses its symbolic nature and the thinker is hurled back into the traumatic Real ("and he would have rediscovered hunger, true hunger"): once he lacks the ability to place hunger in a symbolic register, as a word that carries meaning – the speaker is defenselessly and hopelessly attacked by it.

The biggest task therefore concerns the survival of symbolic language, and the prisoners indeed join forces to ensure exactly that when one evening they organize a poetry reading:

> And from that a language was taking shape that wasn't one of belches and foulness anymore, nor one of dogs yapping around the bucket of seconds. And this language was creating a distance between the men and the muddy, yellow dirt, rendering them distinct from it and no longer buried within it, rendering them masters of it and able also to tear themselves away from the grinding emptiness of their stomachs. In the depths of the mine, in their bent bodies and disfigured faces, the world was opening up.
>
> (pp. 193–194)

As long as language maintains its symbolic quality it has the power to render the one who speaks the master, rather than victim, of his hunger. As long as the word "hunger" doesn't turn into a millstone, into a concrete signified, it can stand between the person and the collapse into the emptiness in his stomach.

In discussing the uncanny aspect of fiction Freud (1919) argues that rather than when the poetic environment is predefined as supernatural (as in fairy tales), the uncanny experience occurs when the artist prevents us from knowing the preconditions on the basis of which he constructed his imagined world, thus confounding the rules of common reality with the rules of a reality that surpasses it. The uncanny environment of the concentration camp precisely and poignantly reflects this definition: an environment whose fundamental assumptions are left unclear: it appears to operate under conditions of "common" reality, based on rituals, a daily routine, a social hierarchy, yet departs from each and every such condition. It is an environment which lacks any experience of accumulation – neither of knowledge, nor of any sort of external or internal orientation. Antelme's struggle is thus for the very possibility to cumulate. This is why he insists to include even the empty holes of thinking in the text. At times, this causes logic to break down, transforming the text itself into a kind of hallucinatory stutter which may only appeal to the reader by allowing it to accumulate within him or her:

> A story. A passion. Away in the distance, a cross. A faint cross, very far away. A beautiful story.
> K. died, and we didn't recognize him.
> Guys died saying, "the bastards, the shits ..."
> The little gypsies at Buchenwald, suffocated like rats.
> M.–L. A.[3] – dead, the hair cut off her head, a skeleton.
> All the ashes upon the soil of Auschwitz.
>
> (Antelme, [1957] 1992, p. 188)

The subject within language, to return to Lacan's (1958), Green's (1988), and Kristeva's (1987) ideas, is willing to lose himself as an actual being in order then to restore himself as a sign, an image, a word, thus bring himself back from death by means of speech. But in the catastrophic reality of the camp speech does not always restore the speaker from death. On the seam line between life and death, speech loses its restorative meaning and power, turning from what hosts the phantom into what is being taken over by it.

As the prisoners are put on a grueling march out of the camp, one of them collapses and is shot dead:

> Two shots behind us. Then only the sound of our footsteps. Everybody heard it; backs remain bent, but the pace quickens. I turned around, but I only saw the road bend out of sight, and the precipice at the edge of the road, and the pines. Who is it? We move a little faster.

> Somebody has fallen. The column moves on. Who is it? In front of us, the SS men have shown no reaction; nobody turns around anymore, and we've already reached the next bend.
>
> (pp. 223–224)

The one thing that interrupts the silent anonymity of the falling man is this look back. Unlike the indifferent men behind and in front of him – Antelme insists on bearing witness to the soundless fall. His turning around isn't just the attempt to find out who it was that fell, but also the recognition of the fact that the erasure of the man who fell is tantamount to the erasure of those who witnessed his fall yet didn't turn around; that when not a trace is left, what disappears along with this trace is the surface on which it might have been imprinted; that a human consciousness that does not register such traces becomes, itself, absent and erased.

> We carried a basket of duralumin together; he said he was from Wuppertal, in the Rhineland. We shook hands on a lovely winter's morning. My life, if it lasts, will always contain that now. I swear this to myself as I walk on with the rest.
>
> (p. 224)

Calling the fallen man's hometown by name, as well as holding the memory of his handshake, mean that although he has been robbed of his life, his death will leave its trace in the memory of the one who witnessed it. Antelme restores the dead man's name and identity from his anonymity. At the same time, in doing so he also turns himself from an anonymous, silenced witness, into a witness who is fully present. In this sense he rescues not only the dead man from the negation of his death: he also saves his own consciousness from its negation through the refusal to bear witness to this death.

> We don't talk. We each try to be ready. Each is afraid for himself, but we have probably never felt such solidarity with each other, never felt so replaceable by absolutely anybody at all. We prepare ourselves. [...] Ready to die – that, I think, we are; ready to be chosen at random for death – no. If the finger designates me, it shall come as a surprise, and my face will become pink [...].
>
> (p. 232)

The difference between "to die" and "to be chosen at random for death" is the difference between having an identity and being anonymous; between owning your death, even if you are not in command of your life, and being robbed even of your death. Being surprised ("If the finger designates me, it shall come as a surprise") is Antelme's defense against anonymity. It is his proof that he is not anyone or no one, but someone – and the blush on his cheeks indicates that for this someone, for this singular being, his death will always be exorbitant – a catastrophe that cannot occur without surprise.

> Yet if he is not to die anonymous, he will have to be reflected, however briefly, in someone else's consciousness; to leave a mark in someone's eyes: It's for those on the sidewalk that we're looking so intently as we go through Wernigerode. We are not asking anything of them; they just have to see us, they mustn't miss us. We make ourselves evident.
> (p. 236)

As the convoy of prisoners moves along, they pass by some buckets which local people have put out on the pavement in front of their houses. Wanting to drink, Antelme approaches one of these buckets:

> When we approach the pails the women get out of the way. One of them stooped to move her pail just as I was bending down to drink. *"Bitte?"* I said and she shook and quickly let go of it. I looked at her – in a natural way, I believe – and then I bent over to take some water. She didn't move; when I straightened up, I nodded slightly to her, but she still didn't budge. So I turned away. In front of this woman I had for a moment behaved like a *normal* man. I couldn't see myself. But I realize that it was the human in me that made her back away. "Please" from one of us, must have had a diabolical sound.
> (p. 244)

This encounter bears out the uncanniness caused by the crossing of worlds that characterizes war situations. As he bends over to drink from the bucket like an animal while simultaneously addressing the woman like a human being, the blend of nonhuman and human makes itself most powerfully present. The woman is paralyzed by this transgression. If he hadn't spoken, she could have thought of him as an animal. If he'd looked human, she could have considered him a man. Could one say that this hybrid creature has resonated something in her, maybe forced her to confront this encounter between the human and nonhuman also within herself?

As the journey proceeds, physical and mental deterioration spiral to the point where the body is no longer experienced in its integrity but as a collection of part objects:

> The first cigarette lights up in the corner near the opening. A mouth pulls on it, and already the next guy's hand has moved up and hovers near the mouth. [...] Now another hand approaches the mouth drawing on the cigarette. It remains suspended and, after the third drag, it tugs at the butt.
>
> (pp. 271–272)

This new language, the subject of whose sentences, rather than a person, is a body part and whose object is an act ostensibly carried out by that body part without the guidance of an intentional mind, illustrates the severity of the narrator's de-subjectivation. It is not merely the body that has been almost completely consumed. Consciousness itself struggles to survive intact. Rather than constituting a center, thinking becomes diffused to peripheral parts in the shape of the body's organs. The loss of center is simultaneously the outcome of this weakness and the reason for its exacerbation. His friends, who are dying one after the other in the train carriage, wallow in their own excrement. The loss of bowel control indicates surrender. Once a person feels he is about to die he stops investing energy into maintaining his humanity. Or perhaps it is the other way around: from the moment a person gives up on his humanity the distance between him and his death grows ever shorter.

Antelme passes the final days of the war in a state of near-death. He is not alone in this. The others, much like him, seem to have lost their outline. They blend into one another, melt into each other's filth, their voices blending into one painful pulp:

> The room is one great throatful of cries and plaints. [...] We are all borne upon a wave that can neither break nor subside into sleep. One cry, one plaint succeeds another. It won't stop.
>
> (p. 280)

As the text approaches its conclusion the narrator loses his "first person singular" to a first person plural, or worse: to an indistinct, disembodied, disappropriated mass of voices. This howling is no longer produced by human beings with distinct names and faces. The wailing seems to be emitted by one body, or by no body at all. The experience is of sounds that erupt from the void left behind these absent bodies.

This is also chillingly borne out by the following lines:

> The man with the bandaged head is getting weaker. Nobody can help him; there's nothing left to be done. [...] He told me yesterday that he used to live in Paris; he was a journalist. I asked him his name.
> "That does not matter anymore," he answered.
>
> (p. 281)

When the American soldiers enter the camp, testifying begins spontaneously:

> The soldier listens at first, but then the guys go on and on, they talk and they talk, and pretty soon the soldier isn't listening anymore. [...] And the prisoner's own experience is revealing itself to him in its entirety, for the first time, and as something almost separate from him. Face to face with the soldier, beyond the reserve he feels he also senses welling up within him a feeling that he is from now on going to be prey to a kind of infinite, untransmittable knowledge. Yet others say along with the soldier, and in the same tone of voice as he, "Yes, it's frightful." [...] Echoing the soldier's expression, they let him think that there is no room for any judgment other than the one he has just made; they let him think that he, the newly arrived soldier, strong and clean, has fairly grasped the whole of this reality, since they themselves, the prisoners, say the same thing he does, in the same tone [...]. And finally, some guys seem to have forgotten everything. They look at the soldier without seeing him.
>
> (p. 289)

One could think of this description as a rough formulation of the various modes of witnessing: There are the excessive witnesses who talk incessantly, their excess keeping their audience at a remove. There are the metonymic witnesses who feel that they are from now on going to be prey to a kind of infinite, untransmittable knowledge. Then there are the metaphoric ones who join in with the listener's language, but while creating a bridge between them and the listener they also lose the full contact with the catastrophe. And finally, there are the *Muselmann* witnesses, the ones who manage to connect neither to themselves nor to the other: unable to appropriate or to convey it, they enact catastrophe as such.

The tragedy of the encounter between the prisoners and their liberators resides in the abyss which the catastrophe has opened up between language – which can only contain what human thinking can perceive – and the experience that puts the victims beyond the pale of what may ever be thought or understood.

> In all this, everything must be believed, but the truth can be more tedious to listen to than some fabulation. Just a piece of the truth would be enough, one example, one idea; but nobody here has only one example to offer, and there's thousands of us. Most consciences are satisfied quickly enough, and need only a few words in order to reach a definitive opinion of the unknowable.
>
> (p. 289)

Antelme points here at one of the most perplexing traps into which testimony can fall, namely that of turning the traumatic object into a saturated one. One characteristic that signals such a saturated object is the "satisfied" conscience, which, as Antelme describes it, "needs no more than a few words in order to reach a definitive opinion of the unknowable". Though Antelme refers to the soldiers who listen to the prisoners' accounts, rather than to the prisoners who gave those accounts, we may assume that there is something in the excessiveness of the accounts themselves – as described before – that contributes both to the listeners' state of mind as well as to the fact that the objects of the account become 'saturated'.

One word that signposts such a saturated state is "Unimaginable":

> *Unimaginable:* a word that doesn't divide, doesn't restrict. The most convenient word. When you walk around with this word as your shield, this word for emptiness, your step becomes better assured, more resolute, your conscience pulls itself together.
>
> (pp. 289–290)

This is the irresolvable catch of traumatized consciousness: Whatever it grasps cannot be held without the grasping consciousness itself being annihilated. So, concepts need to be inserted as buffers between this consciousness and its objects. But the language that achieves this buffering is by definition a pseudo-language: the void from which it arises turns into the chasm into which it very much collapses.

Maybe this is why the one possible human alliance at this point is one that rather than attempting to capture the thing itself encircles the void it has created:

> There's a shadow next to me, and the red tip of a cigarette. From time to time the tip glows brighter, and a mouth and nose are lit up as if by a distant beacon. The ember has moved away from the mouth, which has now been reclaimed by darkness. The ember comes towards me. I am not paying attention. An elbow pokes my arm. The ember gets closer. I take the cigarette, take a couple of drags. A hand takes it back.
>
> "Thanks."
>
> The first word. I'd been alone, and I hadn't even known he existed. Why this cigarette extended in my direction?
>
> I don't know who he is. Again the ember glows before his mouth, then moves away and back towards me. I take a drag. The two of us are together now, he and I: we're taking drags from the same cigarette.
>
> "*Franzose*?
>
> And I answer, *"Ja."*
>
> [...]
>
> In my turn I ask:
>
> "*Rusky*?"
>
> "*Ja.*"
>
> He speaks softly. His voice sounds young. I cannot see him.
>
> *"Wie alt?"* [how old are you?]
>
> *"Achtzehn."* [eighteen]
>
> [...]
>
> Nothing now exists but this man I cannot see. I put my hand on his shoulder.
>
> In a low voice: "*Wir sind frei.*" [We are free.]

He straightens up. He tries to see me. He shakes my hand.
"*Ja.*"

(pp. 292–293)

The quiet, gentle reconstruction of language: from body parts to a whole body, from "mouth and nose" to a hand held out; from where a name no longer carries meaning to where signs of age and origin restore the old concepts of time and space. From chaos, the world is created once more by means of a word, a gaze, the mere touch of a hand.

Notes

1 Originally published in French in 1957 under the title *L'Espèce humaine*. Copyright © 1957 by Editions Gallimard, Paris. First published in English in 1992 by the Marlboro press, Marlboro Vermont. Translation copyright © 1992 by Jeffrey Haight and Annie Mahler. The Marlboro Press/Northwestern edition published 1998 by arrangement with Editions Gallimard. All rights reserved.
2 The "Lyrical Dimension" of the psyche is the dimension that integrates two aspects of the human mind: the "emergent" aspect, which perceives the world, and the self within it, as being in constant flux, as inaccessible to common rules of interpretation and as unpredictable – and the "continuous" aspect, which is responsible for the perception of the world as continuous, predictable and open to explanation in terms of causality, time and space. The lyrical dimension enables us to create a narrative: not merely bear the experience but also store it as a memory (Amir, 2016).
3 He probably refers here to his sister, Marie Louise Antelme.

References

Amir, D. (2014). *Cleft tongue: The language of psychic structures*. London: Karnac Books.

Amir, D. (2016). *On the lyricism of the mind: Psychoanalysis and literature*. London: Routledge.

Antelme, R. ([1957] 1992). *The human race*. (trans: J. Haight and A. Mahler). Marlboro, VT: The Marlboro Press.

Fink, I. (1988). *A scrap of time: And other stories*. (trans: M. Levine and F. Prose). London: Peter Owen Publishers.

Freud, S. ([1919] 1955). The uncanny. In: J. Strachey (Ed.), *The standard edition of the complete psychological works of Sigmund Freud, volume XVII (1917–1919): An infantile neurosis and other works* (pp. 217–256). London: The Hogarth Press and the Institute of Psycho-Analysis.

Green, A. (1988). Preface. In: B. Brusset (Ed.), *Psychanalyse du lien* (pp. i–8). Paris: Centurion.

Kristeva, J. (1987). *Black sun: Depression and melancholia.* (trans: L. S. Roudiez). New York: Columbia University Press.
Lacan, J. ([1958] 2007). *Écrits.* (trans: B. Fink). London: W. W. Norton.
Levi, P. ([1963] 1979). The truce. In: *If this is a man/The truce.* (trans: S. Woolf) Suffolk, UK: Penguin Books.
Ophir, A. (2005). *The order of evil: Toward an ontology of morals.* Cambridge: MIT Press.

Chapter 8

The lacuna

Reading children's testimonies

In his *Remnants of Auschwitz* (2002), Giorgio Agamben mentions that there are two Latin words for the English word *witness*. The first of these is *testis*, whose etymology points at one who puts himself in the position of the mediator or arbitrator, the third party in a conflict between two sides. The other word is *superstes*: the one who is having experienced something to its ultimate end – can testify to it. Based on the movement between the first and the third person of experience, the function of the inner witness (Amir, 2012, 2014) encapsulates both these meanings. In fact, it refers to the ability to shift between being a *superstes* – who has undergone the full experience – and being a *testis* who mediates between the ultimate experience and language. Testimony is always the attempt to bear witness to something that failed to be registered as it happened (Caruth, 1996), and its modalities represent various types of awakening to this failure. In some cases, this awakening takes a metaphorical form, while in others it may take the metonymic, the excessive or the *Muselmann* forms.

This chapter is dedicated to a close reading of testimonies. Some of the testimonies were taken years after the war from Holocaust survivors who had been children during the events,[1] while others were taken from young Holocaust survivors very shortly following the end of the war. Through this variety of texts, I would like to approach the ways in which the traumatic lacuna constitutes language as well as the ways in which language breaks its own rules and generates a syntactic lacuna, opening up an abyss in the very structure of the sentence.

In the close reading of these texts, special attention will be given to breakdowns in their language, assuming that this is the witnesses' way of inserting an experience of ambiguity into the ostensibly coherent flow of speech; the spots where the text's hidden content casts a shadow on its manifest outer layer.

Among the testimonies in question, there will be ones in a predominantly metaphoric mode, as well as ones in which the metonymic and psychotic (excessive and *Muselmann*) modes are more present. Through these variations, I intend to identify and highlight different degrees of reflection and symbolization that enable, respectively, different degrees of healing.

Metonymic repetition, metaphoric deferred action

The testimony of N., born in 1930, revolves around the lacuna that undermines his ability to tell his story. An early example of this lacuna is the memory in which an SS soldier approaches his mother in the street and hits her:

> So then one of them came our way and struck my mother and I remember I was hiding behind ... behind her back, but I don't really remember what I felt. [...] I ... I was a good boy who liked to play and what I remember, what I don't remember, very simply, when it happened there, in the street, I see the picture, I look at the picture and at the boy, I don't feel that it's me inside that boy, I'm disconnected from the boy. The boy sees something there that is not surprising, that doesn't come *out of the blue*, it happens.

This small vignette reflects the intense struggle between the lacuna and the story, between the experience in first person and in third person. Since it is too intolerable to dwell on the first person of experience, a shift occurs to the third person who observes and documents. From this perspective N. does recollect the event and is also able to put it in a logical sequence: "The boy sees something there that is not surprising, that doesn't come *out of the blue*, it happens". But because the third person is not connected to the first person the documentation remains hollow. Language, therefore, breaks down: "... what I remember, what I don't remember [...]". What I remember, in other words, is what I don't remember, and what I don't remember is what I remember – so there's no possibility of telling anything (Amir, 2016, 2017).

This, too, is how he recounts the moment when he and his sister separated from the rest of their family:

> I remember being at an uncle's for some weeks afterwards and then I was told that my big sister, A., and I, we were going to go to Holland and according to the … calendar I figure that I am eight years old, but I didn't really understand at all what it was, Holland. […] What hurts me more is that I do not remember taking leave. A long time ago I asked my sister whether she remembers where we said goodbye – in the street, in the apartment, ah … on the train station, she doesn't recollect, so I don't remember the departure and I miss that.

Shifts in N.'s narrator-position are evident here as well. One moment he is inside the boy, and the next he is wholly outside him, calculating his age only from the calendar. He remembers the general message but cannot remember the exact words, and most of all: he fails to gain access to the concrete, vivid moment of separation: Where did the leave-taking happen, what did they say to him, what did he feel? The pain is not associated with leaving only but also with having failed to register that leaving, which is probably related to the fact that he only realized what was going on a fraction of a moment too late, and thus was doomed, as Cathy Caruth writes, to have never fully known it (Amir, 2017).

Further into the interview he deals in different ways with his dissociation from the boy he was:

> Our parents arrive in Lodz and we send them letters and parcels too. A child understands, one of my painful memories, because I don't have a sense of the boy who does it, we write a letter every so often, to our parents.[…] One of those times I wrote something and I put a bit … ah … of spit on what I have written. So they will understand that I cried. I didn't cry, but I understood they would think I was crying.

Again, there's a shifting between inside and out: the boy doesn't cry, that is, he isn't connected to his pain at that point. But he knows (from his perspective as an observer) that his parents must be thinking that he is in pain, and so he stages the tears which he actually does not shed. The subject of this recollection is thus a double failure (Amir, 2017): that of the adult who does not connect to the child he was ("because I don't have a sense of the boy who does it"), and that of the young boy himself who fails to feel his own pain ("I didn't cry, but I understood they would think I was crying").

N.'s testimony touches also on the experience of the arbitrariness of surviving:

> I mean looking back, I see a chain of ... lucky moments – why two days earlier and not one day later? ... So how will he manage when everything was already locked and when there were loudspeaker announcements every morning that this section or those people must present themselves immediately and ... they were sent away.

The traumatic nature of survival, writes Cathy Caruth (1996), is related to the fact that it is experienced as arbitrary, and thus as meaningless and bearing no relation to the survivors themselves. Survival, too, is a lacuna. In part, N.'s difficulty with experiencing his survival as belonging to him is expressed in his movements between first and third grammatical person, for instance, that from "**I** see a chain of ... lucky moments" to "So how will **he** manage when everything was already locked". Survival remains an estranged, random and alien experience. He doesn't feel it belongs to him in the same way that he doesn't feel that the pain is his. This lacuna, however, is not simply enfolded in the testimonial text: it also structures the latter. We may understand this testimonial act itself as N.'s attempt to re-appropriate his life story and thus to reconstitute an experience of continuity.

> I was hitchhiking without my yellow star and there I am, daydreaming and whistling some tune, there's a man opposite me, he's looking at me, I stop, he goes on singing, and I remember it's a tune from the synagogue. I'm in shock, I tell him, I'm not sure it goes on like that, I heard it from someone, I jump out of my ride, I bolt, because I thought, either he's a Jew or he's a Nazi, how do I know, one has to run away.

How fragile is the bond forged between the boy and the man who sings along with him? The shared song may signal brotherhood, but at the very same time it might be a trap. The same action can signify one thing and its very opposite. In such an arbitrary, random reality, it is no wonder that the most fundamental division between right and wrong, good and evil, enemy and friend, is radically thwarted. The song of the guardian angel and the song of the angel of death may be one and the same song sung by the same person.

In this deep confusion between saviors and assailants, N. recounts how the Dutch people who hid him in their home used to send him out on errands and in doing so endangered his life:

> I remember once when I'm sitting in a train there, and opposite me sits another person, and in my fantasy a conversation starts up – What's your name, I don't know, When were you born, I don't know, What's your father's name, Well, I'll say his name, What's your mother's name, Do you have a brother, a sister, go on, think fast, how old are they. And that's where I go into a panic, I have no story, I don't know who and what to tell that person who … who might investigate me. […] And when I think about it I feel it again, that … that tension […]. And I remember returning home, bringing the things […], I don't dare telling them, 'I have no story'. And they send me off, again and again and … for years, it vanished for many years, but ever since I remembered it I have actually been very angry about how they can do something like that, send out a boy, okay, but without giving him a background story […].

One outcome of a prolonged stay in the territory of the traumatic Real is the attack on the ability to create an uninterrupted narrative, one that is not too arbitrary to serve as a protecting envelope. Having been sent forth into a dangerous world without a "background story"[2] to sheathe him, N. has been abandoned not just by his concrete caretakers – the Dutch people who hid him in their home – but also by the symbolic parental authorities who allowed him to be expelled from his own life narrative into an alienated territory where no continuous and meaningful narrative can exist.

The following paragraph also very clearly renders his attempt to re-appropriate his story:

> One of those moments which I don't … two moments, but one of those moments I want to tell, we were in the street, hunger, cold […], and we hear the Germans' footsteps so we run away, and it seems they saw us, they come running after us. A man [the persecutor] and me. And I, in innocence, totally stupid but that's how it was, I run home. That's what I know. But the house had two entrances, two entrances.

> So I got into one entrance and I ran upstairs to the first floor, [...] and he ran through the ... through the main door, searching, searching, and also running upstairs. And there is this moment when both of us got upstairs, I from my side, he from his, a young guy, no more than 18 or 19 years old, holding a shotgun, and I am sure he sees me. And he does nothing. He turns around and goes away. And I went to that spot several times, and I looked it [sic] from all kinds of angles, whether the ... the sun, the sunlight came in from the window, so it could be that ... the bit in which I am is dark. It might be that the sun came that way, and he had the light in his eyes. Why didn't he shoot me? One of the questions ... the many questions in my life [...] for me that was a very critical moment. [...] I don't understand. Don't know.

The question of why the young German did not shoot him (was it because he didn't see him or because he chose to let him live?) is crucial because it concerns the arbitrariness of N.'s survival. Was it a chance slant of sunlight that left him sufficiently out of sight in that obscure spot – or the sudden compassion of the young German when facing the little boy? Was the fact that he stayed alive mere luck or did it have something to do with who he was? The decision for life remains meaningless and arbitrary: He does not know whether he was saved because the German was momentarily blinded or on the contrary, due to what he saw; and the difference between these two ways of being saved, for him, remains the greatest difference there is. It is the difference between being the hero of the narrative of his rescue and being accidentally and meaninglessly lucky (Amir, 2016, 2017).

N. concludes his testimony with a dream he had after the war ended:

> In the dream I go into our apartment, I'm grown up now, it's our apartment, the way it was. I checked it with my sister and she confirmed. I go into the living room and the air is warm with a fragrance. And I remember it was in our room, that there was some little door there in the middle where we put apples during the winter, to heat them. Then it's not winter, I go into the living room, the whole flat is empty, I go to that chimney, I open the door and there I see four dolls – a father, a mother, and two sisters. And to me this dream is really important because it enabled me to say goodbye to my parents and my sisters.

This dream constitutes an effort to fill the lacuna of his parents' and his two young sisters' deaths in circumstances he didn't fully know for many years. In the dream, he links the moment before separation – the childhood home and the living room – with the end of the story (finding the four dolls in the chimney, which may suggest the crematoria in which his parents' and sisters' dead bodies were burned).

But in addition to connecting between beginning and end, the dream also links between life and death. By inserting into the peaceful living room, with its smell of apples in the oven, the four dolls that represent the dead bodies of his family, he ties the warmth of the living room to the heat of the crematoria, the smell of apples to the smell of charred flesh. Thus, he creates an uncanny domain in which no element remains unambiguous: the smell, the chimney, the warmth: each of them has a double meaning and what appears to generate life proves, retrospectively, to generate death.

This is the irreparable contamination of the world before the rift by the one after it, one in which the living room already carries, with hindsight, the mark of the horror. In this sense, then, the dream does not just deal with the separation from loved childhood figures, but also with the separation from an internal reference to a zone of tenderness, of protection, of the non-ambiguity.

> I learned something during the Holocaust, that [...] you shouldn't take things for what they are. It doesn't cause me to be suspicious. Cautious, yes. But I fear to take it further because then I will depart from the boy inside me. And the boy inside me is very important to me [...] It took me some years to understand that I can give him something, and I still want to keep in him [sic] the boy inside me.

The closer N. approaches the suspicious texture of things the more he risks losing the vital internalized representation of the child he was. Being attracted to having a deep understanding of what he underwent, while at the same time realizing the enormity of the price of such understanding, he leaves intact, incompletely deciphered, the tension between *testis* and *superstes*, the lacuna that constitutes his story and at the same time undermines it.

N.'s mode of testimony is a metaphoric one. It shifts between the vital link to the moment of breakdown and the attempt to reflect on it and render it meaningful. His testimonial narrative illustrates the metaphoric deferred action, the effort to reconstruct his story as a rich continuum beyond its inherent fragmentation. He doesn't adhere to the traumatic memory pictures as static objects, but rather enlivens them retrospectively, transforming the traumatic lacuna from a "negative possession" (Amir, 2012, 2014) which annihilates language into an abyss from which language emerges.

D., born in 1939, begins his story at the moment when his mother smuggles him and his brother out of the window so they won't be caught by the Germans:

> Mother dressed me in a hurry, and ... I even remember that my shoes – she tied carelessly, she didn't ... [becomes emotional] and ... then it was on the first floor. Then we gave ... Mother told us 'You go down', probably she also wanted to get dressed, she was in her pajamas or something I don't know, and we went down and my brother went first, he goes down the stairs, the exit door was exactly next to the stairs. He was about to open the door and my mother from upstairs she shouts 'Don't open the door, for God's sake, don't open the door.' And then she came down, she lifted us in her arms [...], she opened the window and put us through the window. She kissed us and so on and she hugged us [...] and she said 'You go'. Where, where should we go, she said, some farm, you go there, you'll find there [sic], go, ask for help, and so on. We said, 'But don't you want to come with us?', 'No, no, no, no, g-g-go'. The truth is that I don't know whether she said "no no" but she made this movement with her head that she was staying. [...] I thought it was all right, we are going and we will meet mother in some [sic], maybe she'll get dressed, she'll come out and we'll meet her. Because I think she was not dressed, she ... a dressing gown, no more. So I thought we were going to meet her.

This calamity of the separation from his mother is also where his greatest lacuna is located. The childish eyes of the four-year-old boy registered what with metaphorical hindsight he understands was the sign of rupture, the sign that something changed irrevocably: the rush in which his mother dressed him, the fact that she didn't tie his laces in the usual way, her shout not to open the door and her getting them out through the window without following them herself. His awareness, however, could not contain what was happening and so he missed the moment of separation; he did not register the fact that this was separation. This failure, on the one hand, allowed him to escape, but on the other hand never stopped persecuting him as the moment in which he turned away from an event that determined his entire life from then on (Amir, 2017).

> With my mother, the truth is, when she went out shopping or to the village shops, I always wanted to come along with her, I didn't want to leave her, I would … would do anything to get out, she sometimes got out from the window so I wouldn't go with her. I always wanted to be real close to her, to hold her like that, because I also [sic] some sort of fear, they'd already taken my father so I wanted to keep her.

What, then, did it take for this boy, who kept so close to his mother that he never let her leave home without him, to be willing to leave through the window and to walk to a faraway farmhouse, through the forest, with his brother, leaving her behind? Some degree of dissociation was required for him to be able to turn away from her and walk off. Yet alongside this dissociation, there must have been some recognition, even if unconscious, that this is a matter of life and death and that there is no alternative. This ambiguous combination of the greatest possible dissociation along with the clearest recognition of what was going on is what turned the moment of rupture into a lacuna.

André Green (1986) writes:

> In order to survive such unexpected and astonishing desertions of the parents, the child ought to decathexis the remains of his narcissism by turning away from the parents.
>
> (p. 146)

In other words, the dissociation described here constituted a necessary, yet not conscious, act of survival.

One of the most touching recollections in D.'s testimony comes from after liberation, from a forest walk with the woman counsellor of the residential school in which he was then enrolled:

> And I remember one day seeing a family having a picnic, they were eating on the lawn, and I was spellbound, I sat ten meters away from them and I stayed and the counsellor calls, 'Come along,' and so on, I saw … I looked at the family, it was a dream, to see a family, children,

> that's what I remember, one day, like that. And she ... in the end she forced me to go, because I was hypnotized I was ... I sat like that, I was looking at the family and she apologized, she said ... he didn't do anything, I was looking on like that, I saw ...

After D. was separated from his mother, nothing could be, or be perceived as, whole again. Everything concealed the lacuna of her absence, or better yet – the lacuna of his missing the moment of separation from her. The encounter with this intact family, a family which does not hide a lacuna, was an encounter with an impossible world, a world that had long since collapsed within him and which he did not expect to ever encounter again. This is why he looks at the family not only as a memory but also as a dream. In a world whose order turned upside down, exactly this very simple everyday situation contrives to create a sudden experience of uncanniness. Not surprisingly, language, too, metonymically breaks down when he renders account of this scene: Words are repeated ("I looked at the family", "I was looking on like that, I saw"), at several spots sentences don't end at all, testifying to the fact that the encounter with this family takes him back to the moment of rupture, the moment at which the very syntax of his external and internal world broke down and after which reality itself became estranged, forever speaking in a foreign tongue.

Y., born in 1934, tries to figure out the lacuna of the sudden death of her mother who was killed by a shell at the very start of the war:

> We went to sit in the air raid shelter. I remember that I was alone, without my mother, that I remember. I remember the air raid because the lights were turned off, went out, and I remember later it was very difficult to get out of the shelter. That I remember, because to this very day I have problems related to it. I don't like to be in cellars, I feel my breathing stops when I enter caves. All things under the ground make me feel a little like that, uncomfortable. [...] And my mother was injured it seems in many parts of her body because she was covered in blood and I remember that, I remember because there was no one to tell me, my father was not there and my mother died and there were no other relatives. So this I really remember, that I took a handkerchief from someone and I tried to clean the blood off my mother, I kept trying and it welled up again.

The lacuna of the missing moment of separation is prominent here too: the girl is taken to the shelter while her mother is mortally injured, and when she comes out and meets her again she's already bleeding to death and she misses the opportunity to take leave from her. This lacuna of the mother's death is later augmented by the conspiracy of silence with her father and their shared choice not to ever discuss what cut their lives into two:

> Why didn't I sit down and talk with him [her father] about it, that I cannot understand. I could justify it to some extent, but not sufficiently.

The consistent refusal to penetrate the lacuna of not-knowing causes it to grow and expand, taking over more and more regions of consciousness:

> I don't remember what I did, I don't remember, you know, no one asked me, this is the first time, the first time I am asked that I have to think about it and I am not the type of person who asks herself questions, I never did. Never.

The refusal to reconstruct the past, in other words, transforms into an attack on the very ability to produce a continuous narrative. At another point, she tells:

> I remember my aunt, who became blind [during the same air raid that killed her mother], they danced with her, like a tango, that kind of dance, they must have wanted to cheer up those people a bit. Not with my mother, she was in a bad condition, but I remember they danced with my aunt. She died too, what of? I don't know about her injury, other than that she lost her eyesight. I never asked my father about that either, it drives me crazy that I did not ask all these things. [...] But they didn't ask me either, you know, if only someone had asked me [...].

What Y. recounts here offers a partial answer to why it was so hard to "want to know": The image of people dancing the tango holding the injured in their arms creates a site of horror, a site that undermines the very distinction between life and death, between catastrophe and entertainment. This perplexity and the shock resulting from the collapse of all distinctions is itself a massive attack on the ability to think about what happened and to establish it as a memory. In this sense Y.'s testimonial mode is metonymic. Her text remains fragmented, alienated and shrouded in darkness in many places. What is lacking is the perspective of hindsight or reflection. In the absence of a reconstruction of the events, the uncanny experience also lays claim to ostensibly positive memories, like that of the liberation from the camps:

> We got out of the camp and we drove, I remember, in the beginning they went on foot. They walked huge distances with young children, the sick and the old on carts, adults went on foot, this I remember. I remember myself, this is the one thing that has remained a kind of a question mark, whether anything happened to me on that way, because I remember something vague and a little strange, I remember a kind of a beautiful road, and we're on these open carts, big ones, without my father, they went on foot, my uncle and my father and all the people. Something not so clear about what it was there, exactly, something I don't [sic], but something happened. Whether it was good or bad I don't know. [...] I don't know, there's something, it's something. I remember the road being beautiful, fields, green, sun. [...] But there was something there, unclear, during that trip, I don't know what it was.

This text is one big lacuna. On the one hand, it presents a scenario whose details are more or less known: following liberation the children, together with the sick and the elderly, were put on carts, the adults walked, and the journey was headed out of the camp. The primary lacuna, however, keeps perforating the full picture, producing blind zones throughout the entire scene of memory. Y. may delude herself that had she asked herself more questions, or had someone else asked her more questions, she would have been able to join up the details into a proper narrative. But it seems that her narrative is not simply punctured by the missing data or dates, but rather by the fact that what constituted this narrative from the very outset is something she cannot reconstruct, and that therefore returns through the body's symptomatology and through the uncanniness that renders all forms of recollection suspicious, ambiguous and unassimilable.

T., born in 1932, also tells about the lacuna of separation from her parents, when she was handed over to a Christian family:

> At night then when a woman came suddenly whom I didn't know, it was supposed to be ... And I don't recollect how I said goodbye but I remember I must have had a fight with my father because he wanted

> me to put on a coat or something like that and I remember that I must have perhaps left crying, certainly not with a good feeling, but on the other hand this whole thing was not exactly surprising, because they had prepared me, they talked to me about it beforehand that this was going to happen.

Here, too, one observes the oscillations between knowing and not-knowing (Wiseman and Barber, 2008). Though she was prepared for the coming separation, the girl does not know how she took leave. Faintly, she remembers an argument which was disproportionate to such a charged moment (her father died of typhoid shortly after in a labor camp and she never saw him again), she remembers leaving in tears, but she cannot put a finger on the emotional experience of separation.

> I remember how my mother put something around my neck, she put something around my neck, and it seems there were valuable things inside it, maybe rings, maybe things like that, jewellery, in the little bag, maybe cookies, maybe things I loved, I remember having a little bag and this little bag disappeared later on, disappeared, it wasn't with me anymore.

The disappearance of the little bag symbolizes the hole in which everything the girl tried to preserve was lost. Again, we face the lacuna related to the moment where the most important event vanishes into a void which fails to preserve or collect it. There are further manifestations of this lacuna that are related to the form, and not just the content, of reconstruction:

> When we got to that work place, where the Jews worked, the women, she handed me on, someone took me, don't remember who, a woman, and I couldn't get to my mother [...]. And they took me, and either they first bribed the guards, or they said 'Listen we'll hold you on both sides, we'll lift you a little and you'll look taller and you'll look as though you were part of the work team and you'll enter the camp through the gate. And that's how it was. [...] So there, that's the question, what I remember.

The language of this testimony gropes after the event rather than describes it: "and either they first bribed ... or they said" – the narrator herself, that is, does not recollect whether they bribed the guards to smuggle her into the camp, or they made her look taller, or perhaps it was both. She does not know whether what she describes is reality – or whether it is her own attempt to impose a logical narrative on this arbitrary chronology. Often, throughout her testimonial text, the language she uses is a reconstructive-deconstructive one in the sense that she constructs her memory from hindsight while also constantly doubting it:

> To what extent can I repeat today that I remember it this way without relying too much on my diary?

T. is preoccupied by the attempt to distinguish between the memories which she wrote in her diary and the living memories, and she often doubts the emotional vitality of her recollections which seem like a repetition of what she noted down rather than a real vivid recollection. This, too, is a lacuna: one that spreads between what a person has been told, or even what he or she themselves has documented and the living experience they went through. Witnessing narratives often collapse into familiar, worn narratives. What is dropped out of these worn narratives is what was not registered, it would seem, at the very moment of the happening, and therefore cannot be revisited.

This is the case with the following recollection:

> They got us out of the shed and the Germans they told us to march in line and when we passed through the light I saw, there, near the latrines a boy, a friend of mine, he was lying there, injured, dying, and more injured or dying people, and they were begging for help. I didn't know what, no one, us they were taking out in rows and I think it got wiped out, I think I am relying a lot on what I wrote, today, when I try to connect to these images I think I [sic] a great deal was wiped out.

Both form and subject matter here reveal the lacuna from which this account emerges: In formal terms, especially conspicuous is the syntactic fragmentation ("I didn't know what, no one", "I think I [sic] a great deal was wiped out"). In terms of its subject matter, the paragraph tells about a memory which has been robbed, in effect, of its status as memory. This is not because the details it describes did not actually happen, but because the narrator herself does not remember them in a vital manner.

The inability to remember in a vital manner indicates her position as the very event was taking place: the position of one who witnesses something to which she cannot bear witness. Her gaze was turned, at one and the same time, toward the dying boy and away from him, just like it was turned, simultaneously, toward her registering consciousness and away from it. Hence this is not a memory that grew remote but one that was never fully registered.

Further evidence of such a mode of memory-less memory, is manifest here:

> Now they did not allow us either food or drink, I don't think they allowed us to get off the carriage at all, today I am not connected to this recollection. I mean, I think I might remember more from my diary, but I am unable to get linked up to these images of that time, that's what I find strange, because it's rather traumatic, very traumatic. Now when I was thirty I went for treatment with some psychiatrist and there were some rather tough week or two when I was tottering between reality, whether to keep close to reality or to get myself checked into a psychiatric hospital. [...] Now why do I say traumatic, because there was this bit, during my treatment [...], when I was at home, I felt, I went with my husband, that I have to eat, I must eat and I remember telling him in a very hysterical way, and I felt that if I wouldn't eat that very instant, I would die as it were. Today I try to think, to make connections, could I have re-lived it then, during that treatment? At the time, he stopped at some kiosk and bought me a bagel and with that bagel I got to the psychiatrist and it was as though I filled some terrible hole in my stomach. But that was here, when I was thirty, when there was enough food, so I could not have felt such hunger. I think it was related to [...]. Because three days without food?

It is the gulf between the traumatic intensity of the events (hunger, people who suffocate and die due to overcrowding and then are thrown out of the carriage) and the lacuna related to the inability to experience the horror when it happens, that is responsible for metonymically triggering the bodily experience of acute hunger many years later. What was not registered at the moment itself repeatedly left its mark in the course of the years until it found – probably also thanks to the protective conditions of the psychiatric treatment – the strength to break out irrepressibly.

> At certain points in life they would ask me, when I came to Israel, when I still was a girl, and also later when I was a young woman – How come you survived? How come you survived? And that got me wondering too and I started to check why, actually, did I survive, and to evolve all kinds of theories about why I survived. And to this very day, there is no sure answer, but rather all kinds of historical events in whose light I can understand why I survived. So I don't know what to stick to – whether to why did I survive or to what happened, that is, to what are the facts.

As said, the lacuna does not inhere just in the traumatic experience but also in its survival. T.'s attempt to reclaim her survival passes through the "big history", as Perec calls it (in T.'s words: "all kinds of historical events in whose light I can understand why I survived"), but it remains sterile in her personal biography. She does not know why she was saved. This is not because she fails to reproduce the chain of concrete events leading up to it, but because she has no access to the deep meaning of her being saved. The arbitrary nature of her survival, much like that of the trauma itself, together amount to an attack on the ability to feel protected in a world that may be interpreted and predicted. It is no coincidence that language keeps breaking down wherever she touches on moments that cannot be conveyed or understood. This is what happens when she tells about the moment when they brought her to the sauna and crematorium where, eventually, the taps yielded water instead of gas:

> I know that I first entered a sauna and next the crematorium. In the diary it says, what I remember, that they walked us there, today I don't even really remember how it was that water came out, rather than gas as it were. [...] I don't remember. I remember what happened later, facts. Now that you mention it, I think I'm, in a way ... that feelings, apparently, about everything related to the atrocities, that they died, if it's something that is possible, or maybe I repressed it way down and it's better not taken out of there. When you ask what I felt, what I do remember is for instance, a sad story, is that they left some for me some sock [sic], that they put a dress on me, with a small checkered pattern, I must have been given some black and white skirt, because later from that skirt I sewed a bra for my big sister. [...] I don't remember the way we left the sauna [...].

The testimony addressing the moment of near death in fact breaks up twice over: Once, in its language, which becomes fragmented, consisting of half-sentences, conveying bits of information which are put into doubt immediately by means of the statement "I don't remember"; and a second time when the traumatic memory is covered up by another fragmented memory, that of the sock and the dress (skirt?) in which they put her, a memory which serves to bypass the memory that cannot be remembered, a screen memory, a sort of bridge over the traumatic abyss.

> And I don't remember when they did this, I should remember it. I don't even know at which stage in life I decided that I don't remember, I don't want to know this.

At this point the tape recording ends and it seems to have taken some time to start a new tape. When the interview resumes, T. asks: "I am still in Auschwitz, right?"

To testify, for her, is not "to talk about Auschwitz" but "to be in Auschwitz". This is why her language grows more fragmented and truncated as she enters her memories more deeply. This is the broken language of trauma; the broken metonymic language of a child who understands what is going on only partially, only in unconnected segments:

> There are two people who stayed with me, stuck, and don't ask what I felt, don't ask me. I remember on the road [during the death march] someone who was squashed because they had trampled him, I think they squashed him, because it was hundreds, hundreds, thousands of people who were walking, squashed, because his face, as I saw it, was like a fish, something like that. A fish is, fish is something kind of squashed, flattened, that's the word, he was totally flattened, maybe it was a woman, something flat. Because they walked over it. That left an impression on me. And another thing we are walking and some canal [...], I remember water there, there was some figure with his entrails oozing out, and crying, yelling. That's it.

"And those who were on the sides of the road, that wasn't all that impressive", she says elsewhere in her testimony about the people on the death march who collapsed in exhaustion. But, "these two people, the one still because of that flat [sic], the second because of his entrails coming out, that was something". Creating a hierarchy is one way of safeguarding the ability to think. In the absence of the capacity to create such hierarchy, to constitute differences, to put things into categories – thinking cannot occur. In the face of the uncontainable atrocity this child's mind fights for the ability to think, a struggle reflected in the attempt to hierarchically "organize" the horror. This is why she doesn't remember what she felt, yet knows very well what "impressed" her in the procession of the catastrophic spectacle on the roadside. Hierarchical ordering here is not a form of distraction. It is her desperate struggle to preserve consciousness in the face of what is beyond the ability of this consciousness to contain.

At some point she loses her mother for a while:

> My mother wasn't there. And I know I cried a lot, I was inconsolable [...] I lost my mother and that was the end of the story. I didn't want to go on living, it was clear to me. And I don't know, in the morning, perhaps, I went down to pee, God knows what, or resourcefulness, resourcefulness that was quite something, I walked along the orchard and all of a sudden I see my mother. [...] and we found one another and she took me to her carriage, which is where my sister was too. And then she warmed my legs, she took my foot and put my foot, my feet between her breasts and she warmed my legs. That's it. From the moment I found my mother everything else became unimportant, to be with my mother was the most important thing.

"To be with my mother" goes beyond the girl's obvious wish to be close to her mother. "Mother" is the very representation of the good object which when annihilated, as Laub (2005) suggests, releases the by-products of the death drive which the proximity to it neutralizes. Maintaining closeness to the concrete good object allows this girl to preserve a representation of a good object within, one that attenuates the representations of cruelty and evil, one that preserves her ability to conduct an imaginary or concrete dialogue (for instance by means of her diary) with an other, to maintain, that is, a reflective position that transcends the extreme helplessness and makes it possible to transform its excess.

When the interviewer asks T. about her fears she replies:

> Now I have no fears, I have anxieties of a different type, no physical fear. [...] But I remember that I wasn't afraid in the camps either. I do have fears but they're of a very different kind, things that are much less defined and not so conscious. They're vague.

This distinction between fears and vague anxieties is fundamental to the understanding of the traumatic lacuna. Since the most formative memory is not of the kind that is registered and erased, or remembered and repressed, but one that cannot be registered even as it occurs, the associated fears cannot undergo regular processes of condensation, denial, repression or displacement. They rather go on murmuring in consciousness as free-floating, vague derivatives of the empty lacuna, gaining neither meaning nor sensory representation. It can be said that they carry something of the qualities of the lacuna itself: a vague sense of absence instead of presence. One may refer here to Green's (1999) "blank anxiety" as opposed to "red anxiety" (related to injury, destruction – i.e. derivatives of oedipal castration anxiety). This anxiety is marked not by the presence of a horror-inducing object but by the empty space that marks the place in which the latter should have been. The metonymical mode of T.'s testimony is the enactment of this empty space in language. It reports not through words but through the empty spaces between them; not through the links it generates but through their fragmentation. Even when this testimonial text includes explicit memories they do not retrospectively absorb meaning, but rather stay in the same crude mode in which they were captured in the first place. They serve not as an expression of a developed point of view – but rather as a repetition of the moment in which the narrator herself has turned away.

A., born in 1934, was separated from her family when she was six:

> This silence inside ... First in the middle of the night and in the house, I didn't understand and I asked where my mother was. And my father said my mother felt unwell, she was taken to hospital, and while she was in hospital we would be with the women [two unfamiliar women the girl sees for the first time in their home], and when she would feel better we'd return home. And my big brother, he was already nearly 15, he was terribly sad. [...] And he gave me a book, to put in my pocket, or I don't know, I was holding it. He gave me a book.

A.'s testimonial narrative preserves the perspective of the little girl throughout, without "strayings" to the adult viewpoint or to explanations with hindsight for the benefit of the listener. Preserving a clear metonymic testimonial mode, A. takes the listener on a journey which fits the size of the girl she was, bringing to life the sense of disconnection, fragmentation, helplessness and horror she herself experienced at the time. The book her brother put into her hands, the book which, she repeats twice, he gave her, is not just a kind of "transitional object" (Winnicott, 1971). It serves as a thread connecting between the first part of her childhood narrative and the other part that is about to start now. This thread is so crucial to her because the reality after the rupture, which began that night when she was taken to an unknown institution, is characterized by an attack on any ability to link between what happens from now on and her previous life:

> I'm given a chain with an identity number and I ask where I am, I ask the nurse where I am. (sighs) It's hard. She tells me I am an abandoned girl, she tells me I am an abandoned girl, and I don't know what that is. And then she senses I don't know what that is, and then she explains very thoroughly and says that I will never see, neither my father nor my mother, and I ask 'And where are my little brother and sister?' and she says my siblings, too, I won't see. I am an abandoned child, my father and mother don't want me anymore and that's it. The shock I felt I cannot … It's hard for me to understand what happened to me. It's clear that I was shocked but I cannot put any feeling to that word. It's as though it wasn't me. As though it wasn't, it was a mistake, it wasn't me.

So the rupture is not merely what cuts between life as it was and as it will be from now on. It is the total breakdown of biographical and emotional continuity. The girl has not only been robbed of her previous life, in her family, with her parents; she has also been deprived of the ability to render meaningful the terrible loss she experiences. The statement "you are an abandoned girl" erases not only the future ("that I will never see, neither my father nor my mother") but also the past. It is a statement that perpetrates an all-out and cruel attack against the girl's ability to keep a sense of sanity, actually creating a psychotic reality in which whatever has been so far loses its truth value, becoming instead a kind of lie or fiction in a way that makes it hard for her to distinguish between reality and dream and between hers and not hers ("It's as though it wasn't me").

> I remember I started reading in the book and they came to take the book away. That is to say, now I have nothing. I no longer have my clothes, I no longer have my book, I have nothing. I, simply, as I say, and I don't think I am mistaken, I am no longer me. It's really no longer me.

Meanwhile this girl conducts a terrifying struggle against this alienation, taking position by the door to the dormitory for hours on end in order to catch sight of her small brother and sister from whom she was separated:

> And I stood at the door to see whether I could see my brother and sister, [...] and that's how I stood near the wall without budging but I saw nothing. For how long I stayed there I don't remember. I feel it was a long long long time. Many days, maybe many weeks, maybe many months, I don't remember, just a feeling of it being a long long long time.

The fact that A.'s testimonial narrative does not adjust itself to her retrospective knowledge that this first separation from her siblings lasted only five days, attests to the metonymical nature of her testimonial text. The time of trauma is experienced as an eternal present, unchanging, with neither a link to a past nor a connection to a future. Stern (2004), along with Modell, introduced the concepts of kairos and chronos into the psychoanalytic thinking. While kairos is the Greek term for human cyclical, nonlinear time, the kind of time that can turn back on itself in ways that allow meanings to change and grow – chronos is the "scientific" or objective, linear time, which does not allow the future to affect the past. "Unless meaning is embedded in kairos – that is, unless experience can move freely between the past, present, and future – new meaning cannot come into being. [...] In kairos, we circle back on our histories in ways that are routinely nonlinear and cyclical, and sometimes also capacious, endless, and oceanic. It is precisely this embeddedness in the fertile ground of kairos that trauma steals from us" (Stern, 2012, p. 57). In other words, the time of trauma is neither kairos nor chronos. It is circular in a non-creative way. It lacks both its simple, objective, common linearity as well as its oceanic fertility. This alienated aspect of time is a central component of the uncanniness that is so typical of the traumatic experience.

In A.'s testimony such an uncanny moment of encounter occurs when she does not recognize her siblings after she finally meets with them:

> The cart is empty and the women who are with us tell the younger children to sit in the cart, and she tells me to look after the children, they have to deal with the tickets, I don't know. [...] And all the children start to cry. All of them. And I don't know what to do. And I face the children and tell them not to cry and not to cry and suddenly I see a boy (sighs) who isn't crying. He doesn't cry. He looks at me with a frightening expression, big eyes, a frightening expression, and I look, look (sighs) and I say 'K' [her little brother's name] and he responds with a look 'I don't understand' and I see it is K. He knows his name. Because I feel he responds to me, to that name. [...]. And I say 'K.', and I say, look at that child, he isn't crying, he isn't crying. And I approach him and I want to take him, and he sits and suddenly I see another girl who doesn't cry, and I look and look, and I need a very long time to know that I am not wrong and I say 'N.' [her little sister's name], and N. responds to her name, with her eyes. And I know that I have been waiting so long, I was on the same minivan with them, I looked at all the children and I did not recognize them.

This is an appalling moment. The brother and sister she was looking for all that time appeared before her very eyes and she did not recognize them. She failed to identify them not because they had physically changed (as said, she was only separated from them for five days) but because they belonged in the world before the rupture, a world from which her present is severed not merely in terms of place and time but also in terms of meaning. Like her, they, too, did not recognize her (although the fact that they were the only two children who didn't cry implies that they somehow identified her as their older sister, even if not consciously). They stared at her as though they'd seen a ghost, and she too experienced them like two little ghosts, half belonging to the present world half to the one that was lost. This is the experience of the uncanny at its most intense: where the familiar and the alien are welded together, creating a terrifying, disastrous ambiguity.

A few moments after reuniting, the children are once more divided:

> The suffering a child might undergo because it is not strong and has no protection, it cannot do anything and all I wanted was to hold them and protect them [...] and that was for me, I think, there is no word to explain that suffering. It is suffering, it is a huge cry that is stifled in the throat and cannot get out and it is also a pain in the stomach, there's no right word to explain. It's the worst I experienced in my life, when my brother and sister left me. I watched them as they left, until I saw that tiny spot and they were gone. [...] I thought, worse than that, nothing [sic], it cannot get.

Their second disappearance, after she already found them, was even more traumatic than the first. It was the silent, terrible confirmation of the fact that there was no end to the catastrophe, and in that sense it was not only taking place now but would go on forever.

Throughout the years she spent in the village with her adoptive family who raised her as an abandoned child without knowing anything about her and while she herself didn't know anything about this only being a cover story – A., who read books from age four, understood nothing of what she was taught at school and inexplicably and consistently failed in all subjects:

> And I go on going to school, while I understand nothing, I kept getting zero, zero, zero, and only in church I feel well. In church I learn everything. I understand everything and I go on hating Jews. And in this way three and a half years went by. That's a lot of time. Three and a half years is a huge amount of time to learn and understand nothing, like you don't learn anything and to go to church and to think about what the Jews did to Jesus. I mean, with me everything is the other way around. Instead of thinking that the Jews were wretched, for me it was all the other way around, to think about the Jews that killed a small child, I don't think about the adult, I only think about the child, I find it terribly hard. Three and a half years passed and the war ended. [...] When I returned to F. [her home town] everything came back [i.e. her capacity to learn]. Everything apparently went on without me noticing, but I was unable to answer questions, I couldn't take tests, all I wanted was to read, only to read, but I had no books.

In order to survive, the girl had to adopt the narrative that was imposed on her from outside, a narrative according to which her parents abandoned her. She consciously takes in this narrative while constantly, underneath it, murmuring the opposite narrative for which she unconsciously struggles. Hence, she has to cope with an ongoing clash and ambiguity which cause an arbitrary tear in her emotional and identity narrative. This tear attacks her ability to think and thereby prevents her from learning and internalizing any new material. Underlying the ambiguous psychotic narrative there is a constant prohibition to think and to know (Amir, 2010, 2014). This prohibition does not only concern the one thought she is not allowed to think ("I am a Jew") but along with it every other thought that might remind her of that thought or somehow connect to it. This is how the prohibition on a thought transforms into a comprehensive prohibition on thinking.

Especially interesting in the context of this testimonial text is the report that the desire to read is the only area in which her curiosity remains intact. Perhaps it was related to the fact that the last thread connecting her to the previous world was the book that her brother had given her when they parted. Reading, in that sense, may have connected her unconsciously to what her conscious mind was forbidden to connect to. Perhaps it also had to do with the fact that reading pulled her away from the concrete reality, which subjects such as mathematics, physics and geography in which she constantly failed – confronted her with. One can think of the general rules of perception and causality, represented by these subjects, as contradicting this girl's inner experience of a lack of any ability to understand the world in terms of sequence and meaning.

It comes as no surprise that she fears she might never grow up:

> The fear is because I cannot know more than I know when I don't understand what interests me, I am always at the same level so when I'll grow up I'll stay at the same [sic], like a girl, like a fool. Which means I'll never be an adult. I don't rise, I simply stay in the same place. When I'll be 30 or 40 years old, that's what I think, I'll be speaking at the same level, I won't know more.

The fear of not growing up is associated both with the frozen traumatic present and with the prohibition to gain access to the forbidden narrative, which in the case of this girl became translated into an injunction against any growth, emotional or intellectual. Interestingly and shockingly, this prohibition on knowing is reproduced when she is found again by her father at the end of the war:

> And when I wanted to tell my father, nevertheless, what happened in the village, he said 'Be quiet, you should be grateful, you're alive [...]'. That's all I heard. And next he very quickly got married to a very young woman whose parents went to Auschwitz as well as her sister and her brother and all the pictures were up on the walls and they would say 'You see, you see, that's what could have happened to you like them in the gas chambers, you must not tell.' And I felt, because I felt so much hatred toward me, so I said Memer [the woman who took care of her in the village during the war] was right, the Jews are not nice, those Jews, I hate them, and I continued praying to Jesus at night. [...] My father only cared for one thing – to know what happened to his parents and his brothers and he knew there was no chance, as far as he had heard, that any of them would return. What about my story, he has no patience to listen [...]. It's as though one isn't allowed to live. And so I wanted to die.

The prohibition on telling her story was experienced as a prohibition on life itself. She was found but no one took an interest in her. Her story came full circle as it were when she was finally told that she was taken to the institution in an effort to rescue her, not to abandon her, but in fact, she was now abandoned for the second time into the ambiguous reality in which her father, who had struggled so hard to find her, turned out to be alienated from her, her siblings treated her as a stranger and the people around her made her feel guilty for staying alive when so many others had perished. Again her ability to create a continuity of experience came under attack. This time the prohibition on thinking did not originate outside but inside the home. This prohibition constituted a second undermining of her ability to think, causing her to identify with the aggressor as a result: to identify with the hatred of Jews (who were now attacking her in the shape of her closest relatives) and with the wish to annihilate them – to the point of wishing to annihilate herself as well.

Many years later, married with two adolescent children, she decides to board a ship to Haifa. For her, this is an act of reparation:

> Four in the morning, it is very very cold, and we are in Haifa, in view of Mount Carmel, the sun, it's so hard for me to tell, is starting to rise.

> I look at the sky and the sun and I can't speak and I only think, I've got these thoughts racing fast through my head, you see, you're safe [...]. And I think of my grandfather and grandmother whom I never knew, both my grandmothers, my mother, my aunt and cousin, all of whom perished in the gas chambers [...]. All of their faces come back to me and they are, as it were, with me [...].

Her insistence to move away from the traumatic zone allows her to restore the generational continuity ("All of their faces come back to me") and herself as part of it. For the first time since the age of six the traumatic temporality may be replaced with regular temporality, one which links the dimension of the past with that of the present, producing thereby the possibility of a future.

The empty grammar

The testimonies considered in this section are a selection from the protocols of 55 accounts by children, archived in the Warsaw Jewish Historical Institute (Elstein, 2014). The close-reading will focus here on those testimonies whose style was obviously excessive, matching what Cathy Caruth (1996) has called "empty grammar": an attempted reconstruction of the event which in fact erases it. Empty grammar, too, is evidence of a lacuna. It comes to mask the inability to know by means of "over-knowing" which takes hostage, as we will see, both witness and listener.

The account of Lea Goldberg (born 1929) is exemplary of this type of testimony:

> I was living with my sister, brother and mother in Rafalovka, when the murderers, the Germans, took over our city, and when I saw them I said to my mother: "I cannot bear to look at them. I want to live, I am young, I cannot look on as the German murderers torture us, I must get through this and take revenge on these criminals". A whole year went by, full of troubles, hunger, contempt ... Then suddenly one lovely summer's day, SS people arrived and sealed the city and everybody got ready to die. I was 12 years old. I go to my mother and I say: "Mummy, let's go, let's escape, let's not go like lambs to the slaughter". I kiss my mother: "I want to live, come on let's escape, let's escape!"
>
> (p. 68)

In a note to this text, the editor mentions that the witness is unlikely to have been familiar with the expression *like lambs to the slaughter* at the time of these events and probably inserted it in her above-cited words after encountering it following liberation. This inclusion after-the-fact is in fact typical of her general tendency towards esthetic augmentation. This esthetic augmentation, which marks her testimony throughout, transforms the traumatic object into a saturated one, whose descriptive excess actually blocks the possibility to retrospectively think it anew. The expression *like lambs to the slaughter* does not evince rich metaphoric usage, in that sense, but rather pours the personal experience into a given format while blocking the authentic link with it.

> On that day the German murderers shot all our dear ones. And my dear mother, and my sister and my brother, they fell victim there to such a very tragic death. I am alone, I have no one, I am alone like a stone. That's how I went along, hungry, alone, and broken.
>
> (p. 69)

The use of intensifiers ("such a very tragic death"), images ("I am alone like a stone") and repetitions ("I am alone, I have no one, I am alone like a stone"), along with the use of direct quotation (adding both a dramatic and melodramatic effect) all add up to a testimonial syntax that overcompensates for the experiential void by means of excessive description. The result of this esthetic augmentation is an effect of saturation. Failing to deliver the catastrophe vividly, the excessive testimonial narrative captures it in a kind of rhetorical splint.

These saturated descriptions also characterize the portrayal of her flight through the fields and her knocking on the door of the person who eventually saved her:

> When the doctor returned, I tell him: I don't want to stay here any longer. I must escape, stay alive and take revenge on the criminals who tortured our dear mothers, our fathers, sisters, children, and brothers. I am running away … I must live … As soon as the sun set and everyone was in their beds I jumped out of the window in my pajamas and escaped. I ran through swamps, through the forest and the field, and I reached my dear Uncle. I knocked on the window and called out: "Daddy, open, save me, it's me, Lola!" He came running, we started to cry, kiss […]
>
> (p. 71)

Further on she tells:

> They tortured those whom they burned alive. One day they brought a Polish man, fifty years old, they cut his belly, tore out part of his entrails and tied him to a tree, and two Banderovci paraded him around until they took out all of his entrails. They stuffed children's mouths with potatoes until they suffocated. [...] Jewish children, they would kill them with knives, slash them. I saw all this with my very eyes. It was horrible, impossible.
>
> (p. 71)

The statement "I saw all this with my very eyes", repeated throughout her testimony, aims to ensure that the listener will feel no doubt. Facing the impossibility of the events she describes, events that exceed any psyche's capacity to contain, certainly that of a child, she wants to underscore the reliability of her witness position. However, this attempt to bolster her witness position does not relate merely to the doubt that might arise in the potential listener. It also reflects the gap from which this testimony arises from the start: the gap between the incapacity to contain the traumatic events and the attempt to nevertheless capture them in a well-constructed narrative. The phrase "I saw all this with my very eyes" thus comes to cover the traumatic lacuna into which facts are sucked until they lose their liveliness, turning into saturated, frozen, fixed objects. This saturation is covered by pathos, as in the closing sentence of her testimony:

> My dear ones! Take revenge on the criminals who took away all hopes, all of life's dreams. Take revenge! Revenge!
>
> (p. 72)

The account of Dora Hazan (born 1928) also forcefully evinces the use of the excessive testimonial mode:

> On 16 August 1942, Lutsk was taken to the slaughter. The ghetto organized resistance. The revolt went on for two weeks until it was gagged. And the rebels, in the flashlights of movie cameras, were forced to jump into the river, naked ... injured ...
>
> (p. 164)

The very first words of this quote already install the rhetoric of excess. The statement "Lutsk was taken to the slaughter", turning the town of Lutsk into a human subject, is not a factual description. The act of turning the town into a subject taken to the slaughter stretches the limits of suffering from a collection of individual persons to an immeasurable generality. The sentence "and the rebels, in the flashlights of movie cameras, were forced to jump into the river, naked", too, exceeds factual description. The witness' awareness of the film cameras (whether as concrete objects or as an image) symbolically renders her awareness of an audience witnessing the spectacle of her testimony and of her dramatic effect on them. As in the previous example, here, too, the testimonial narrative uses dramatic and theatrical dialogues throughout, achieving a dramatic effect by building up a lively tension. Thus, the witness does not only convey the details of the event but also presents a lively rendering of the horror. As a result, the traumatic event is usurped by "the story of the traumatic event", while the witness stays trapped inside.

> I remember that evening as one of the most horrible moments in my whole life. I got used to the 'rations', the heat, the examinations, the prisoners. And suddenly I find myself expelled from paradise into the bleeding, cruel, and murderous world. Naked, barefoot, hungry, and alone – Where is one to go? W-h-e-r-e? – But because I knew it was forbidden to linger too long, dreaming near the prison, I ran to the nearest church … Already twice, the beadle was going to lock the House of God, but when he saw a girl bathing in tears, tears made of blood, he went up to the priest.
>
> (p. 166)

The repeated use of imagery referring to bodily secretions ("the bleeding, cruel, and murderous world", "a girl bathing in tears, tears made of blood"); the amplification of suffering by means of the split account of detention as "paradise" (as opposed to the inferno into which she was set free); the repeated question "Where is one to go? W-h-e-r-e?", suggesting that "W-h-e-r-e?" reaches far beyond the concrete question – all of these together draw out, almost by force, the melodramatic effect, as though to express that the details alone will not convey the intensity of her real suffering.

An especially interesting moment in this testimony occurs when she tells about her escape, back to the convent, in the middle of prayers:

> After six months of 'sanctity and purification' they took me to a church to say the evening prayers. When I kneeled down, I noticed one of our neighbors giving me a terrible look and really wanting to swallow me with her green eyes … Because I knew that things could become dangerous, I immediately got up and quickly went to the convent. After this 'prayer' the nun turned to me in anger:
> 'What did you do?'
> I tried to explain:
> 'I had a heart attack!'
> She slapped me in the face and threw me out and at daybreak she betrayed me to the priest.
>
> (pp. 166–167)

In more than one sense it would have been possible, and even better, to mention anything else (belly ache, stomach upset, period) as an excuse for her disappearance from prayers. But the reference to a heart attack is not arbitrary: on the one hand, it bears out the excessiveness, the need to amplify and augment which, it would seem, marks not merely Dora's testimonial style but also her personality style. But on the other hand, it also exposes her lack of capacity for transformation of excess: for in fact, her experience, on noticing one of her former neighbors in the prayer room, was much closer to being a heart attack than a stomach ache. The fact that she opted for the thing itself – rather than an adjusted version of it – indicates her inability to convert the excess of anxiety. This is why her testimony, in spite of its obvious rhetorical quality, remains trapped in the register of the Real.

A further illustration of this inability to convert excess occurs in the description of how she emerges from hiding in the monastery and faces the Soviet liberators:

> I told the nuns:
> 'I'm going out to see the Soviets!'
> The nuns looked at me, puzzled:
> 'Renee?'

> 'Let me out, I'm a Jew!'
> 'What's come over you? Are you crazy? You're a Jew? Ha ha ha ha.'

That laughter made me angry and I opened the door wide:

> 'I am a Jew. I am the one Jew left out of 24,000. I must go and welcome the liberators of Europe who have restored my right to exist!'
> When I saw the first tank I took hold of the heavy chains, some captain lifted me up, I fainted.
>
> (p. 167)

Her fainting in the arms of the captain expresses inconvertible excess which instead evacuates itself through the body. This however is not just the accumulated excess of traumatic events, but also the product of what Cathy Caruth (1996) called the "awakening" from them and toward them. This awakening itself involves a traumatic effect, one that embraces both the missed encounter with the catastrophe as well as the incomprehensibility of survival. As a result of this awakening, this witness steps up the intensity more and more, to the point of overflowing the limits of her own psychic container.

The testimony of Charlotte Perlmutter (born 1929 or 1930) is especially interesting with regard to the above two testimonies, due to its shifting from a position of verbal excess to a wordless state.

Her testimony starts, as do the other two, with a dramatic and melodramatic description:

> When I saw that black bacchanalia in our town, during the first weeks of the occupation, the Jews being hit, abused, raped, shot – I left my girl friends and I stopped talking to people. I made a very serious effort to learn the German language. For days and nights on end I read, wrote, recited poems, talked to myself in German. [...] My parents, my older sister, and brother suffered tremendously. After four months of studies I started on my way with a small suitcase and I said goodbye, 'ashamed', to all my loved ones [some unclear words], my darkening birthplace.
>
> (p. 276)

Her immediate response, in the face of the traumatic events, consists of a withdrawal from her familiar world as well as from her mother tongue.

This withdrawal into herself is not only documented in her descriptions but also enacted in so far as the speaker avoids direct reference to concrete events and instead only offers a theatrical version of them.

Like the two earlier accounts, this one too employs direct dialogue:

> A German car drove past. I raised my hand impertinently:
> 'Stop!'
> The car stopped and a German man shouted:
> 'Who are you?'
> 'A German!'
> 'What's your name?'
> 'Charlotte!'
> 'Where are you from?'
> 'Vannet, Brennet' – lit: From where it burns.
> 'I must get to Lokachi right now!'
> 'Get in!'
>
> (p. 276)

The many exclamation marks give one some idea of the dramatic mood generated by this girl's witness account which offers a lively staging of what happened to her – as if she was starring in a play rather than as if this play was actually written on her own flesh and blood. Her sudden departure from the rules of grammar in what she says next, quite conspicuous given her general articulateness, discloses what has not come through:

> On the way **I** told them about my parents' tragedy. How they were murdered by criminals. **She** herself escaped through the window. It's been eight days since **she**'s left Germany, to 'rough Ukraine', and still **she** hasn't found a place …
>
> (p. 277, emphasis added)

The transition from first to third person (a transition the translator specifically marks as hers in the original), signals, by means of the collapse of grammar, the failure to experience, let alone report, the traumatic event in the first person. The grammatical rupture, however, also enacts the traumatic event to which it testifies, since the result of it is that she becomes alienated (as expressed in the use of the third person) from herself and her identity – as indeed is about to happen in reality.

> When the city started bleeding. When Lutsk was destroyed, when my sisters and brothers fought heroically for two weeks, were killed and thrown into the river – I lamented my fate pretending I had a toothache … I worked at their place until they fled the city and with them …

Here the interviewer adds:

> She had no more words. She wept.
>
> (ibid.)

This testimony moves, as Agamben (2002) suggests, between either having a voice but nothing to say – or having a lot to say but no voice. The collapse into wordlessness does not merely mark the collapse of the excessive mode, but also the moment when the emergent true emotional connection makes this excessive mode superfluous. This is why the empty grammar of excess disappears the moment she regains her cry.

The return of the ghost

In a paper entitled "Psychiatry, Testimony and Shoa: Reconstructing the Narratives of the Muted" (Greenwald, Ben-Ari, Strous and Laub, 2006), the authors claim that out of 5000 long-term psychiatric patients hospitalized in Israel since 1999, a disproportionate number of about 725 were identified as Holocaust survivors (p. 245). A review of these cases showed that these patients had not been treated as a unique group and that their "trauma-related illnesses" had been neglected in their decades-long treatment. Most of these patients had been diagnosed as having chronic schizophrenia, with no special attention given to the historical circumstances related to their psychiatric symptoms and disabilities. The psychiatrists who treated them frequently insisted that these patients did not respond to traditional treatment such as antipsychotic medication (p. 246).

I believe that the Muselmann psychotic mode reflects exactly those states of "trauma-related illnesses" which create a chronic-psychotic picture, untreatable by traditional means (Amir, 2016). The following illustration describes such a case.

During my work in a psychiatric hospital, many years ago, I treated P., an Auschwitz child survivor. She was more or less of the same age group as the interviewees mentioned before. But in her case, the lacuna turned into the story itself.

"Clothes", she would repeat as she pointed at the photograph of her mother whose murder she apparently had witnessed. "Clothes" – and she would try to tear her hospital clothes from her body and run naked into the shower room. Only later did I learn that that's how she had last seen her mother: naked, as she was being kicked in her belly and head, and taken, along with other women, into the gas chambers. The word "clothes" for her pointed not at an object or an image but at a situation. It did not take her back into the past but resurrected that past actively, yet in a dissociated manner, in the very present.

There was something else that P. repeated over and over, not a word but a musical sequence made up of broken syllables. Assuming this was a sort of psychotic mumbling, the staff allowed her to repeat this endlessly without trying to find out to what it might refer. But one day, P.'s sister came for a visit and when P. started the sequence again, the doctors asked her what it could mean. The sister broke into tears and told them that the sequence was a code which she and P. had memorized throughout their years in Auschwitz just in case they would manage to escape. Their mother had taught them this code which was made up of letters representing the names and telephone numbers of people who had promised to help them and take them into their homes. To ensure that little P. would remember, her mother had put the code to music and sang it to her as a lullaby. The song was all P. was left with from her mother and she continued humming it to herself long after the mother was no longer alive.

When P. emerged from Auschwitz she was almost starved to death. She had lost the ability to speak, refused to eat and was in a catatonic state leading to many psychiatric hospitalizations throughout the years. The only two verbal signals she salvaged from this annihilation of language and thinking were the words that resurrected the last moments of her mother, and the syllable combination that signaled the continuity that was interrupted when her mother died: the continuity between past and future (the people who promised to hide them were former friends of her parents), the continuity between the world before the rupture – a full world in which promises were kept and relations were maintained – and the empty world that came after it.

Primo Levi writes (1989):

> The destruction brought to an end, the job completed, was not told by anyone, just as no one ever returned to describe his own death.
>
> (p. 84)

P. did not return to describe her own death: it was her death that returned in her shape. What remained of that little girl were not the remnants of her personality as it had been, but rather the space surrounding who she could have, but never would, become. She herself became the lacuna undermining her story along with the possibility of telling any story ever again.

The struggle of these witness-children is the struggle to gain entry into what Agamben (2002) calls "the archive of statements", without losing the link between what is stated and what cannot be uttered out loud. The act of testimony is always one of simultaneously waking from the nightmare and waking into it, one of capturing the event and losing hold of it, one of turning history into a personal narrative and of the collapse of that personal narrative into the historical unknown. But counter to what one might expect, the traumatic lacuna is not silent. It has black-hole like qualities: it engulfs, it ensnarls, in its emptiness it is a sounding box for infernal voices. One might listen to this lacuna as one listens to the sounds coming from a seashell. Like the shell, the lacuna is a space saturated by the traces of what is not there; it is the ultimate signifier of the encounter between the moment of missing the actual scream and the resonance that will forever range beyond it.

Notes

1 These testimonies were taken from the Ray D. Wolf Centre for Study of Psychological Stress, University of Haifa, Israel.

2 The fact that N. chose the combination "background story" instead of the more common "cover story" may also be telling: it is the background that he most prominently lacks.

References

Agamben, G. (2002). *Remnants of Auschwitz: The witness and the archive.* (trans: D. Heller-Roazen). New York, NY: Zone Books.

Amir, D. (2010). The split between voice and meaning: The dual function of psychotic syntax. *International Forum of Psychoanalysis*, 19(1), 34–42.

Amir, D. (2012). The inner witness. *International Journal of Psycho-Analysis*, 93, 879–896.
Amir, D. (2014). *Cleft tongue: The language of psychic structures*. London: Karnac Books.
Amir, D. (2016). When language meets the traumatic lacuna: The metaphoric, the metonymic and the psychotic modes of testimony. *Psychoanalytic Inquiry*, 36(8), 620–632.
Amir, D. (2017). Traumatic miss and the work of mourning. *fort da*, 23(2), 7–16.
Caruth, C. (1996). *Unclaimed experience: Trauma narrative and history*. Baltimore, MD: Johns Hopkins University Press.
Elstein, H. (2014). *Yaldei ha-milchama 1944–1948: Yeladim mesaprim al ha-shoa*. [The children of the war 1944–1948: Children telling about the Holocaust]. Tel Aviv, Israel: Books in the Attic.
Green, A. (1986). The analyst, symbolization, and absence in the analytic setting. In: *On private madness*. London: Hogarth Press.
Green, A. ([1993] 1999). *The work of the negative*. (trans: A. Weller). London: Free Association Books.
Greenwald, B., Ben-Ari, O., Strous, R. D. and Laub, D. (2006). Psychiatry, testimony and shoa: Reconstructing the narratives of the muted. *Social Work in Health Care*, 43, 199–214.
Laub, D. (2005). Traumatic shutdown of narrative and symbolization. *Contemporary Psychoanalysis*, 41, 307–326.
Levi, P. (1989). *The drowned and the saved*. (trans: R. Rosenthal). New York: Vintage Books.
Stern, D. B. (2004). The eye sees itself: dissociation, enactment, and the achievement of conflict. *Contemporary Psychoanalysis*, 40, 197–237.
Stern, D. B. (2012). Witnessing across time: Accessing the present from the past and the past from the present. *Psychoanalytic Quarterly*, 81, 53–81.
Winnicott, D. W. (1971). *Playing and reality*. New York: Basic Books.
Wiseman, H. and Barber, J. P. (2008). *Echoes of the trauma: Relational themes and emotions in children of Holocaust survivors*. Cambridge: Cambridge University Press.

Chapter 9

Modes of memory, modes of healing

Language is not merely an act in the symbolic order. It is a form of expression in action. The four modes of testimony to which this book is dedicated are, thus, four expressions in action, each producing its own path towards the traumatic object and away from it. The metonymic mode creates a language whose action is repetition; the language of the excessive mode issues in stagnating action; the *Muselmann* mode creates a language marked by evacuation, while the language typical of the metaphorical mode results in deferred action (Amir, 2016).

These actions represent four modes of memory: Repetitive memory, which preserves the link to the traumatic object merely by the apparent motion of repetition but without the possibility to contemplate on it; excessive memory, which keeps the traumatic object frozen in a rhetorical formaldehyde, thus enacting a double, paradoxical movement of preserving it while also preventing vivid access to it; *Muselmann* memory which renders the traumatic object present by means of its repeated negation, and metaphoric memory which dynamically recreates the traumatic object by means of the back and forth movement of thinking (Amir, 2016).

In this context it is important to distinguish between modes of objectal memory versus modes of negative memory:

The metaphoric and metonymic modes are modes of objectal memory in the sense that they maintain memory as a present object that allows processing (in the case of the metaphoric mode) or repetition (in the case of the metonymic mode). The excessive and the *Muselmann* modes, by contrast, dwell in the domain of negative (blank) memory, and thus constitute two types of object negation: one by means of a recurrent act of evacuation, and the other through a recurrent act of stagnation. Of these two types, the excessive mode is the most beguiling: its subtle rhetoric creates the illusion of a present object but simultaneously negates it as a living one. Unlike the phenomenon of repression, which concerns a living object even if there is no conscious access to it – in the case of the excessive testimonial mode, rather than being repressed, the traumatic object is stagnated. It is not buried alive (which would also allow it to be extracted) but kept in a preservative solution that does not allow it to undergo transformation, not even in retrospect.

Gampel and Mazor (2004) write in this context:

> These are things that are not repressed. They are sometimes present through suppression, where though there is no neurotic prohibition, impossibility exists. When the possibility to make a representation or evocation exists, a certain distance must be kept. If there is no distance, nothing can rise to the surface, and the representation becomes impossible.
>
> (p. 547)

Bion (1970), through his notion of the *container contained* interaction, pointed at three possible types of interaction he called *symbiotic, commensal* and *parasitic*:

> I shall not trouble with the commensal relationship: the two sides coexist and the existence of each can be seen to be harmless to the other. In the symbiotic relationship there is a confrontation and the result is growth producing though that growth may not be discerned without some difficulty. In the parasitic relationship, the product of the association is something that destroys both parties to the association.
>
> (p. 78)

Continuing his ideas, it seems possible to formulate these three types of interaction also in relation to the interaction between the remembering subject and the traumatic object. One could think of the metonymic mode of memory as expressing a *commensal* interaction, an interaction which involves an interdependency that allows for the survival of both the remembering subject and the traumatic object but in a manner that may impede further development.

On the same lines, one can consider the excessive and the *Muselmann* modes of memory as expressions of a *parasitic* interaction, in which both the remembering subject and the traumatic object are annihilated. In the *Muselmann* mode the traumatic object becomes a negative possession which annihilates not only itself qua testimonial object but also the remembering subject qua witness, as is clearly seen in the case of P. described in the previous chapter. In the excessive mode, however, *jouissance* fixates the traumatic object in a saturated state which stops all psychic movement to and from it, preserving thereby both itself and the remembering subject in a state of inertia. Finally, the metaphoric mode may be considered to render a *symbiotic* interaction between subject and traumatic object in the sense of enabling the subject to turn the traumatic memory into a psychic possession, and thereby to absorb new associations and undergo transformation. Memory, in the metaphoric mode, acts in a way that can be likened to the work of the dream: much like the dream narrative, the memory text creates symbolic distortions, forms connections whose meaning is hard to trace back, presents facts that disguise and camouflage themselves – all in the service of the simultaneous deconstruction and reconstruction of the traumatic object. The modes of blank memory, by contrast, do not enable memory work in the same manner as psychotic states do not enable dream work (Amir, 2016).

Green (1999) writes a lot about what happens when the subject's capacity to represent the primal scene, which is the source of his being, is obstructed. One can refer to the traumatic object as the force that annihilates the subject's capacity to create a representation of his or her own origin, and thus prevents the experience of a valid and meaningful existence. Constant negation, thus, is the subject's way of marking the formative event: when the primal scene cannot be represented – the inability to represent becomes the subject's very essence, and negation becomes her or his only way to be.

References

Amir, D. (2016). When language meets the traumatic lacuna: The metaphoric, the metonymic and the psychotic modes of testimony. *Psychoanalytic Inquiry*, 36(8), 620–632.

Bion, W. (1970). *Attention and interpretation*. London: Tavistock.

Gampel, Y. and Mazor, A. (2004). Intimacy and family links of adults who were children during the Shoa: Multi-faceted mutations of the traumatic encapsulations. *Free Associations*, 11(4), 556–568.

Green, A. ([1993] 1999). *The work of the negative.* (trans: A. Weller). London: Free Association Books.

Chapter 10

Awakening the narrator

Clinical work with modes of testimony

Trauma is not only the destruction of signifieds: it is the destruction of signifiers. It is not about the death of the good ones or the triumph of evil, but about the catastrophic collapse of the signifier "good" and the signifier "evil", along with the collapse of the distinction between them. If the catastrophic fusion of signifiers is the illness, then treatment would consist of the recovery of these signifiers and the reinstatement of the differences between them (Amir, 2016a).

Hanna Segal (1987), in her paper "Silence is the Real Crime", writes that the atomic annihilation destroys the possibility of symbolic survival, unlike normal death or even death during a conventional war that preserves the symbolic idea of survival after and beyond one's concrete death (p. 7). The struggle for the creation of a testimonial narrative is therefore not about the restoration of the concrete order, but about the restoration of the symbolic order which had been destroyed.

One of the questions that must be considered in working with traumatic memories is how the various modes of witnessing emerge in the analytic interaction, and in what way the analytic interaction can be leveraged as a transformative force that helps shifting from one mode of witnessing to another. The analyst's active psychic space is one of the key parameters in facilitating movement from one mode of testimony to another. But for this to happen, the analyst must present himself as an active container in the face of the traumatic object: not a passive receptacle of traumatic contents (Anzieu, 1989) but rather an active container which performs a transformation of his own in relation to the contents deposited in him, using various forms of *reverie*, projective identification and alpha function (Bion, 1967).

Active containing will never take the shape of a ready-made interpretation, externally imposed, but rather of a complex modeling of thinking processes in which the analyst fights the obliterating force of the traumatic object which is wielded through the transference, evolving a counter-movement between the various modes of counter-transference responding to it.

The various chapters of this book have illustrated various modes of such active and passive containing of the traumatic object. Assuming that the various literary works, as well as the witness accounts, can be listened to in ways similar to testimonial texts delivered in the analytic session – a crucial attention must be paid to the question when does it occur, as we observed in Ka-Tzetnik's book, that the secondary characters hold the inner potential for survival. How can one distinguish, as in Perec's work, between real and fictional memories and which one of them holds the deepest truth? When, as in Agota Kristóf's work, does the use of the third person plural negate the narrating I? And, finally, when does the "awakening" of testimony become a collapse into "a dream that cannot be dreamt" (Ogden, 2003), as in Appelfeld's and in some of Ida Fink's stories, and when, as in Antelme's work, does it constitute the narrator not only as the dreamer of the dream, but also as "the dreamer who makes the dream understandable" (Grotstein, 2000)?

Analytic work with trauma may collapse into each of these modes: it may collapse into repetition, into stagnation, into evacuation. Each of these modes carries its own danger: while the danger of the metonymical repetition dwells in the refusal of reflection and the danger of the *Muselmann* psychotic evacuation lies in the massive attack it creates on thinking, the risk of the excessive mode is related to the fact that it may generate what I call "pseudo-analysis", using its sophisticated rhetoric to preserve stagnation.

Chana Ullman (2014) writes:

> In the treatment of survivors, the witnessing other transforms the silence and absence to a loss that can be mourned. While absence represents the mythical that is indescribable, loss represents the real. Placing the mythical in the realm of the real historical and biographical time makes it possible to mourn.
>
> (p. 442)

In light of this observation, it is possible to reframe the distinction between the excessive and the *Muselmann* modes, on one hand, and the metonymic and the metaphoric modes, on the other, as the distinction between modes that preserve the mythical status of the traumatic object versus modes that situate it in the realm of the real, in the historical and biographical time. Analytic work with trauma may collapse into the mythical position which gives the traumatic event an infinite quality (irreducible to thinking and language), or else encourage the capacity of the subject to place the traumatic memories in a finite biographical context and thereby enable the crucial work of mourning.

The focus of the analytic and psychotherapeutic work with testimonial modes must therefore address form no less than content, language no less than the objects it describes. Survivors' narratives will tend to pull in the direction of content, not just because the content has a powerful (and intimidating) pull – but also because it is easier to focus on the external massive happenings than on the internal "stage directions" which are used in order to reconstruct those happenings. And so psychoanalytic treatment should be looking for the stage directions, for the mode of reconstruction no less – and sometimes even more – than for the details of the reconstructed scene. Since every traumatic testimonial narrative contains a combination of all four modes with various shifts between them, it is extremely important to identify the singular combination of modes that characterizes each narrative, focusing on the specific zones in which a shift occurs from one mode to another. Such an interpretational focus is crucial to the rehabilitation of the psychic metabolic system which conditions the digestion of the traumatic materials, allowing a metaphoric working through of traumatic zones that so far have been only accessible to repetition or evacuation.

The current chapter focuses on the creation of hermetic narratives (Amir, 2016b) in the course of the analytic treatment. The term "hermetic narrative" refers to a condition in which an excessive, hermetically sealed narrative of witnessing is jointly created by the analytic dyad. This narrative becomes an addictive and subjugating object in itself, which while reconstructing the victim-aggressor relations both within the individual and in the analytic relationship – may create what I call "false analysis": an analysis which is based on the malignant cooperation of the analyst and patient with the internalized traumatic object.

The horror evoked in the psychoanalytic work with traumatic memories is not related to the re-enactment of the traumatic experience itself, but to the demand of the analytic situation that the subject would rethink this experience over and over again, ask questions about it, understand it from various distances and angles, digest it in a different manner each time and allow new associations to be absorbed in it.

Traumatic memories have the tendency to barricade and isolate themselves from all other memories. As a result, living aspects of the self can never flow towards them or form an associative link with them. Because of the fear that the new memories would become "infected" with the traumatic ones (and also vice versa – the fear that the traumatic memories will be touched by common life materials) – the psyche creates in some cases a hermetic isolation wall which prevents access to the traumatic memories. In that way, they continue to dwell within the mind as sequences of facts – but it is extremely difficult to create a vivid movement to or from them, and to transform them by means of such a movement from solid to flexible psychic matter. This isolation puts the traumatic narrative into a kind of psychic formalin jar which preserves it as a coherent sequence at the cost of retaining its static and frozen state. A "pseudo-access" to the traumatic contents thus takes shape: on the one hand, a tight and convincing testimonial narrative is preserved; on the other hand, this convincing narrative has a double role: it simultaneously preserves the story while withholding any vivid access to it (Amir, 2016b).

The analytic work with traumatic zones is disturbing and unsettling for the subject not only due to the contact with the intolerable contents of his or her traumatic experience – but also due to the fact that it involves the unsettling of the very subject who had undergone these experiences and now bears witness to them. In order to avoid this unsettling blow, an ostensible witnessing narrative is erected as a hermetic defensive wall, preventing all contact with the traumatic materials instead of paving a way to them. This obstructed, hermetic narrative is characterized by a number of recurrent properties:

The first such property is the fact that it repeats excessively, usually in the same exact manner, including moments of hesitation, outbursts of emotion and moments of evident "recalling". In fact, there is a sense that the "story" takes over the narrator's place, becoming a kind of tyrant to whom the narrator is subjugated rather than vice versa.

The second quality typical of these narratives is the massive use of splitting mechanisms. These mechanisms denote a dichotomous division of the story protagonists into demons and victims, as well as a dichotomous division of the narrator's own life experience into the former wholeness and the subsequent oblivion, often with the purpose of holding the subject protected in the position of "the sublime witness" (Goldberg, 2007) or the "sublime victim" (Amir, 2016b).

The third property typical of these narratives is that they impose a recurring feeling of totality and a "life or death" sense of urgency – while the hidden objective is to deprive both narrator and listener of a free reflective space.

Finally, the fourth and salient property of these narratives is their constant refusal to all sorts of interventions. Any attempt to inquire, to observe from a different angle, to question the absoluteness of the narrative – is either repulsed or ignored. The listener (in this case – the analyst) is in fact a captive audience, an audience that is convened for the purpose of passively validating the narrative merely by its presence; a muted audience, of which the narrative effectively demands to erase itself as a subject and to become, instead, an object at the service of the story. This can be understood as a variance of the primary traumatic event itself: the victim, who in his past had been forced to surrender his subjectivity and become hostage at the service of the perpetrator – becomes himself the one who, by means of his testimonial narrative, now forces his listeners to surrender as thinking subjects, turning them into passive extras in a theatre play in which they have no voluntary role (Amir, 2016b).

This happening has profound implications in relation to the analytic process. In order to maintain the powerful status-quo described above and to preserve the traumatic object in a static and unchanging state – it is actually required to withhold any vivid link between patient and analyst, allowing only a pseudo-connection to take place. This is often expressed by a total identification of the analyst with the patient, an identification which may be accompanied, at least for a period of time, with admiration and glorification of the patient's powers. In fact, the analyst is erased through this identification as a separate subject, losing his ability to let the contents deposited in him undergo any transformation.

In practice this often manifests as an experience of paralysis: an inability of the analyst, reflecting the inability of the patient, to tell the story from more than one perspective or to let the patient's enactments undergo processes of reflection and introspection in the transference-countertransference relationships. This is, in fact, a covert and deluding enactment of the terror of the internalized traumatic object on both analyst and patient: as a result of this terror, the patient pushes the traumatic materials into the analyst's "throat" in such way that the analyst is no longer capable of digesting them and can only spew them back out or leave them stuck as they are. Analysis fails in this case in one of its most important tasks, which is to extract out of the trauma's saturated component the unsaturated one, allowing for rethinking and change. In that way, both the narrative itself and the cooperating analyst turn into a mechanism for the conservation and recycling of the traumatic object. This paradoxical defense mechanism is a defense against the psychotic aspects of the traumatic reality – which had turned into a psychotic reality itself: Disguised as an attempt to map reality – it actually projects its inner contents on that reality, painting it with its own colors. Anything that does not validate the story as it is – becomes excluded, while whatever validates it is swallowed without digestion (Amir, 2016b).

Analysis which takes this form is often experienced, at least in the beginning, as allegedly successful, one in which the patient feels understood and the analyst feels as if taking part in a highly meaningful happening. Yet underneath the seemingly ideal surface, a vacuum resides. Unless recognized and interpreted – this mechanism might constitute a pseudo-analysis in which both partners are unconsciously and painfully trapped.

This formalin-like, hermetic state is a state of pseudo-liveliness. Its notable advantage is its power to create a semblance of solidity, of coherence and un-equivocality. In contrast, the living state is far less absolute, far less self-assured, far less stable. It is a state of constant liability, of continuous modulations in the experience of security and in the sense of validity. The patients who produce those hermetic excessive narratives are dreadfully fearful exactly of this living state, since it unsettles their confidence in their own witnessing narrative, and even more since it might resurrect the pain that the formalin-like state has succeeded to nullify. In that sense, they have an immense interest not to allow that living state to ever be generated.

At the same time, however, they possess an equal measure of hope, conscious or unconscious, that analysis will release them from this rhetorical and emotional formalin into a true, vivid, relationship with an-other. It is exactly this hope that the analyst may drop while surrendering to the delusional rhetoric of the hermetic excessive narrative. The importance of avoiding the collaboration with this terror-inflicting mode is related to the fact that the erasure of the analyst as a subject not only recreates an inverted variation of the original traumatic scene, but also revalidates it as an infinite perpetual state within which it is possible to shift between the pole of the victim and the pole of the perpetrator – but impossible to break free (Amir, 2016b).

If one of the main features of the traumatic state is stagnation – the most determined fight against this stagnation is the attempt to create movement in relation to traumatic memories. There are different levels of movement in this context, as we have witnessed throughout the various chapters of this book: alongside highly developed ones there are movements characterized by regression and repetition. But each and every one of them is preferable to the lack of movement produced and preserved by the excessive hermetic narrative, where the narrator is enslaved to the story while the inner witness is paralyzed or anesthetized.

To work with trauma is to awaken the narrator. Not just to grant him a voice – but to insist on this voice's necessary hesitant, stuttered quality – a quality which constitutes the only chance to enable true liveliness where there were so far only artificial substitutes for life (Amir, 2016b).

In "The Work of the Negative" (1999), Green describes "the fertility of the negative" (p. 187) as a creative force that takes place only in the form of negation. This alludes to what occupies the very core of the analytic work with trauma: the possibility of turning negation from a black hole into a space (Amir, 2016a); the capacity of transforming the repeated awakening to the nightmare of trauma into an act of creation, one that extracts from chaos a world in which hell itself speaks forth, thus becoming language.

References

Amir, D. (2016a). When language meets the traumatic lacuna: The metaphoric, the metonymic and the psychotic modes of testimony. *Psychoanalytic Inquiry*, 36(8), 620–632.

Amir, D. (2016b). Hermetic narratives and false analysis: A unique variant of the mechanism of identification with the aggressor. *Psychoanalytic Review*, 103(4), 539–549.

Anzieu, D. (1989). *The skin ego*. (trans: C. Turner). New Haven and London: Yale University Press.

Bion, W. (1967). *Second thoughts*. London: W. Heinemann Medical Books.

Goldberg, A. (2007). "The era of the witness". A lecture given at the Scholion Centre, The Hebrew University.

Grotstein, J. S. (2000). *Who is the dreamer who dreams the dream?: A study of psychic presences.* Hillside, NJ: The Analytic Press.

Ogden, T. H. (2003). On not being able to dream. *International Journal of Psycho-Analysis*, 84, 17–30.

Segal, H. (1987). Silence is the real crime. *International Review of Psycho-Analysis*, 14, 3–12.

Ullman, C. (2014). Introduction to panel: Dissociation, enactment and collective trauma: The role of psychoanalysis. *Psychoanalytic Dialogues*, 24(4), 441–443.

Epilogue

Hiroshima Mon Amour and the command of boundary violation

The plot of the film *Hiroshima Mon Amour* (Marguerite Duras and Alain Resnais, 1959) unfolds in Hiroshima during the summer of 1957. A French woman, married, in her thirties, arrives to play in a film about peace. On the eve of her return to France, she meets a Japanese architect, married himself, with whom she has a short affair. While the affair takes a banal course, typical of such rushed encounters, the fact that it takes place in Hiroshima attaches a shade of disaster to each and every nuance of the narrative. The woman and the man are not mentioned by name throughout the film, we know them as "She" and "He". "What Are they talking about?" asks Marguerite Duras, at the opening of her screenplay. "About Hiroshima. [...] One can talk about Hiroshima anywhere, even in a hotel bed, during a chance, an adulterous love affair. [...] What is really sacrilegious, if anything is, is Hiroshima itself" (Duras, 1960, pp. 8–9).

In the course of their long conversation, it emerges that the woman had a German lover in 1944 – and he died. When this love affair became public, the people of her town shaved her head to punish her for disgracing her fatherland, and her parents locked her up in the cellar of their house in Nevers. And so, her personal trauma is set off in the screenplay against the collective trauma of Hiroshima. They are neither made to compete nor are they put side by side for comparison. Like the man and the woman who represent them, they simply exist, creating a conversation throughout the screenplay in various and complex ways. The affair between the French woman and the Japanese man happens outside time and space, and simultaneously, at all times and in all places. This absolute detachment which coincides with an absolute connectedness is reflected in the final scene when they name one another:

She: Hi-ro-shi-ma. Hi-ro-shi-ma. That's your name.
He: That's my name. Yes. Your name is Nevers. Ne-vers-in France.
(p. 83)

Duras, writes Nurit Peled Elhanan in her epilogue to the Hebrew translation, believed that to imprison words in syntax was to deprive them of their suggestive power. For Duras, the words that count most are the ones which we look for and cannot find. To see means to see nothing; to speak is to say nothing, and oblivion is the one thing we can remember.

He: You saw nothing in Hiroshima. Nothing.
She: I saw everything. Everything.
(pp. 17–18)

She: [...] I didn't make anything up.
He: You made it *all* up.
(pp. 17–18)

In a chapter entitled "Literature and the Enactment of Memory" (1996), Cathy Caruth proposes that *Hiroshima Mon Amour* is "a story of a telling" (Caruth, p. 27). Her argument is that the film asks how can we avoid the necessary betrayal of the particular past by its understanding. Resnais and Duras, argues Caruth, believed paradoxically that the specificity of history could be communicated only through a fictive story, not one *about* Hiroshima but one that takes place *in* it. Thus, the traumatic narrative encapsulates a fundamental paradox: For the Frenchwoman "Hiroshima", rather than the event that brought suffering upon the Japanese, is the event which spelled the end to France's suffering. What meant the "end" for the French, was the beginning of the Japanese ordeal. And so the narrative of French history annuls the narrative of Japanese history by swallowing it and imposing its own meaning on it (ibid., p. 27).

Obviously, the self-same contradiction is part of the structure of the Frenchwoman's story too: For her, the day when France was liberated from the German enemy was the day that her lover was executed. So she, too, carries this same paradox that entangles one's private narrative of suffering with an other's narrative of liberation from suffering. Caruth suggests that the madness attacking the woman – due to which her parents lock her up in the cellar – is actually her attempt to hold on to the event of her lover's death and to her faithfulness to the dead lover. Her refusal to be taken up by the general liberation narrative expresses itself in the damage she does to her own body as the sounds of the French national anthem penetrate her prison from the street. Her refusal to see or to understand is her way of maintaining the link to the catastrophe through the body. It is no coincidence, writes Caruth, that the healing of her hands, the re-growth of her hair, as well as the return of her ability to see – are linked to betrayal:

> I am beginning to see.
> I remember having already seen before – before – when we
> Were in love [...].
> I remember.
> I see the ink.
> I see the daylight.
> I see my life. Your death.
> My life that goes on. Your death that goes on.
>
> (p. 63)

Thus, Caruth claims, the woman's own inner dynamic movement towards sanity functions as a form of betrayal. In order to be "reasonable", in order to recover, she must stop her mad clinging to the memory of her dead lover. But resigning her madness is tantamount to betraying her past – requiring as it does a willingness to be assumed into the collective narrative and temporality – into the history of the others.

"I told our story", says the Frenchwoman to her German lover. "I was unfaithful to you tonight with this stranger. I told our story. It was, you see, a story that could be told" (p. 73). How can testimony be an act of transmission rather than betrayal? How can the act of passing on the story to another person– something that naturally implies understanding – exist as an act that does not simply and by definition annul the catastrophe?

If the singular nature of the story is to survive the act of testimony, its irreducible quality must be retained not just by way of thinking but outside thinking as well. For this to happen, a singular language must come into being between addressor and addressee – one whereby the singular narrative is not submerged in the narrative of the other. This language can be conceived of as an act of hospitality[1]: the hosting of the horror by the physical and mental digestive system of the story's addressee. What this hosting implies is that transmission or communication does not occur through the host's thinking but as a result of the attack which the act of testimony perpetrates on body and mind and of the addressee's very ability to name and connect. Unlike projective identification, where materials which the person is unable to digest are deposited in the addressee so that he digests them on the person's behalf – here it is a matter of hosting whatever resists digestion by its very nature: what the act of digestion itself destroys. This resembles the ventriloquist's voice that issues from the body of a doll. The doll does not serve as a digestive conduit. It functions as a kind of vessel, an amplifier, a sound system. The addressor's foremost request from the story's addressee is to agree to host inside her or himself the horror's voice without ingesting it into the latter's system of thinking. To let it sound its voice in its full, singular exposure, arbitrary and raw.

This is why the Frenchwoman does not tell her Japanese lover "about" her German lover and instead turns to the former as if he were the latter, resurrecting in this way, in the present between them, both his life and death:

> When you are in the cellar, am I dead? asks the Japanese man.
>
> (p. 54)

On the one hand, as Caruth has mentioned, the very question presumes a distinction between the time of the living and the time of the dead. On the other hand, the question is posed in the voice of the dead man as he speaks through the living man – and who, in the course of the story, becomes her dead lover to whom she addresses the story of his death. This blending of times and voices, of the living and the dead, illustrates how the violation of boundaries is resurrected in the scene of witnessing. Only when the living person transforms into a living-dead one, and the dead person becomes a dead-alive one, the collapse of the story's boundaries comes to life in the act of testimony: a collapse which is in fact the one thing the woman wants to recount. For what she tries to share with the Japanese man is not the death of her lover as such, but rather the way she has been robbed of the possibility to know the moment of that death – as a result of which she has also been prevented from fully knowing her own life.

Emanuelle Riva, who played the Frenchwoman in the film, revealed in an interview a fascinating detail (Caruth, 1996, p. 50): The actor who played the Japanese man did not know French at all and was therefore simply reproducing meaningless sounds throughout the various scenes. In terms of the present discussion, we might think of this as a kind of phonetic "hosting" of a meaningless text to which the actor lends his voice. In this act of reciting, he cancels out himself by way of an interpreter – or a thinker – and lends himself as a sound-box in order, thus, to fully deliver this film's testimonial text. This rendition is full exactly because it is void of meaning, because it is a pure rendition of sound, of the voice's fragments. This is the double injunction of hospitality that characterizes the position of the addressee in the testimonial scene: To offer oneself as a sound box to the raw sounds of testimony while not blending them with one's own understanding – yet simultaneously hold them as a thought; to attach oneself to the sound which the story itself produces as if it were imposed from outside, in all of its arbitrariness – and yet as though it emerged from one's deepest core.

To some extent, this is reminiscent of our first impression of the sound-object of infancy. This is a voice whose one meaning is its meaninglessness, and which may gradually gain significance related to its specific rhythm and texture only if we are ready to host it. Like the primal object, trauma demands absolute hospitality in a way that it precedes all meaning. At the basis of this hospitality is the declared willingness to take into the mind's and body's reaches what exceeds knowledge, and to forfeit the entirety of the internal space for its sake before turning it into a thought, before drawing it as a memory, before shaping it into a single word.

Note

1 Jacques Derrida (2000) coined the term "Hostipitality" which combines "hospitality", a word of a troubled Latin origin, with "hostility" – its very contradiction that is incorporated into it.

References

Caruth, C. (1996). *Unclaimed experience: Trauma narrative and history*. Baltimore, MD: Johns Hopkins University Press.

Derrida, J. (2000). *Of hospitality*. (trans: R. Bowlby). Palo Alto, CA: Stanford University Press.

Duras, M. (1960). *Hiroshima mon amour*. (trans: R. Seaver). New York: Grove Press.

Index